Michael Scarce

Smearing the Queer
Medical Bias
in the Health Care of Gay Men

Pre-publication
REVIEWS,
COMMENTARIES,
EVALUATIONS . . .

"I have been and continue to be impressed by the scope and depth of Michael Scarce's observations and articulation. . . . The continued effort to educate health care professionals to this fundamental reality is revitalized by his writing."

Robert E. Penn, MBA
Author, *The Gay Men's Wellness Guide*

"S *mearing the Queer* is just what the doctor ordered—or should. A work of subtle analysis and great originality, this display of what's antigay in the health sciences manages also to be a funny, sexy, moving and, above all, necessary guide to the future of gay men's health. Scarce is a visionary."

Walter Armstrong
Editor in Chief,
POZ magazine

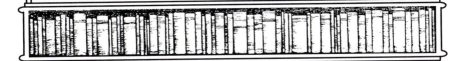

The Haworth Press, Inc.

Smearing the Queer
Medical Bias
in the Health Care of Gay Men

HAWORTH Gay & Lesbian Studies
John P. De Cecco, PhD
Editor in Chief

The Bear Book: Readings in the History and Evolution of a Gay Male Subculture edited by Les Wright

Youths Living with HIV: Self-Evident Truths by G. Cajetan Luna

Growth and Intimacy for Gay Men: A Workbook by Christopher J. Alexander

Our Families, Our Values: Snapshots of Queer Kinship edited by Robert E. Goss and Amy Adams Squire Strongheart

Gay/Lesbian/Bisexual/Transgender Public Policy Issues: A Citizen's and Administrator's Guide to the New Cultural Struggle edited by Wallace Swan

Rough News, Daring Views: 1950s' Pioneer Gay Press Journalism by Jim Kepner

Family Secrets: Gay Sons—A Mother's Story by Jean M. Baker

Twenty Million New Customers: Understanding Gay Men's Consumer Behavior by Steven M. Kates

The Empress Is a Man: Stories from the Life of José Sarria by Michael R. Gorman

Acts of Disclosure: The Coming-Out Process of Contemporary Gay Men by Marc E. Vargo

Queer Kids: The Challenges and Promise for Lesbian, Gay, and Bisexual Youth by Robert E. Owens

Looking Queer: Body Image and Identity in Lesbian, Gay, Bisexual, and Transgender Communities edited by Dawn Atkins

Love and Anger: Essays on AIDS, Activism, and Politics by Peter F. Cohen

Dry Bones Breathe: Gay Men Creating Post-AIDS Identities and Cultures by Eric Rofes

Lila's House: Male Prostitution in Latin America by Jacobo Schifter

A Consumer's Guide to Male Hustlers by Joseph Itiel

Trailblazers: Profiles of America's Gay and Lesbian Elected Officials by Kenneth E. Yeager

Rarely Pure and Never Simple: Selected Essays by Scott O'Hara

Navigating Differences: Friendships Between Gay and Straight Men by Jammie Price

In the Pink: The Making of Successful Gay- and Lesbian-Owned Businesses by Sue Levin

Behold the Man: The Hype and Selling of Male Beauty in Media and Culture by Edisol Wayne Dotson

Untold Millions: Secret Truths About Marketing to Gay and Lesbian Consumers by Grant Lukenbill

It's a Queer World: Deviant Adventures in Pop Culture by Mark Simpson

In Your Face: Stories from the Lives of Queer Youth by Mary L. Gray

Military Trade by Steven Zeeland

Longtime Companions: Autobiographies of Gay Male Fidelity by Alfred Lees and Ronald Nelson

From Toads to Queens: Transvestism in a Latin American Setting by Jacobo Schifter

The Construction of Attitudes Toward Lesbians and Gay Men edited by Lynn Pardie and Tracy Luchetta

Lesbian Epiphanies: Women Coming Out in Later Life by Karol L. Jensen

Smearing the Queer: Medical Bias in the Health Care of Gay Men by Michael Scarce

Macho Love: Sex Behind Bars in Central America by Jacobo Schifter

When It's Time to Leave Your Lover: A Guide for Gay Men by Neil Kaminsky

Strategic Sex: Why They Won't Keep It in the Bedroom by D. Travers Scott

One of the Boys: Masculinity, Homophobia, and Modern Manhood by David Plummer

Homosexual Rites of Passage: A Road to Visibility and Validation by Marie Mohler

Smearing the Queer
Medical Bias
in the Health Care of Gay Men

Michael Scarce

The Haworth Press
New York • London • Oxford

The Haworth Press, Inc., 10 Alice Street, Binghamton, NY 13904-1580

Cover art by Linda Howard.

Cover design by Monica L. Seifert.

Library of Congress Cataloging-in-Publication Data

Scarce, Michael
    Smearing the queer : medical bias in the health care of gay men / Michael Scarce.
      p.   cm.
    Includes bibliographical references and index.
    ISBN 0-7890-0410-0
    1. Gay men—Medical care. 2. Heterosexism. I. Title.
RA564.9.H65S28 1999
362.1′086′64—dc21
                                                                 99-23095
                                                                    CIP

This book is dedicated to Matt Brown

ABOUT THE AUTHOR

Michael Scarce is a doctoral student in medical sociology and Coordinator of Lesbian, Gay, Bisexual, and Transgender Resources at the University of California, San Francisco. Serving as a national consultant and lecturer on sexual health, he is also the author of *Male on Male Rape: The Hidden Toll of Stigma and Shame.* His work has appeared in publications such as the *Journal of Homosexuality, Journal of American College Health, POZ* magazine, and *Diseased Pariah News.*

CONTENTS

SECTION IV: CLEARING THE SMEAR

Foreword

Eric Rofes

I hunger for informed, thoughtful writing about gay men's health issues. When a book is published about gay men's mental health, medical issues, addictions, or sexualities, I bolt to the nearest independent bookstore, track down the volume and eagerly leaf through its pages. My hands frequently tremble with anticipation.

More often than not, I find myself deeply disappointed. Our bodies, health needs, and erotic lives usually are discussed in superficial ways. Writers—including gay male writers—bring profound moralistic judgments to their discussions of gay men's cultural and sexual practices. A decade of these visits to bookstores had turned my hunger into starvation.

When I seek out materials on women's health—including lesbian health—I have a different experience. Often their literature is sophisticated, politicized, and informed by cross-disciplinary approaches to gender and the body. The writing is nuanced, respectful of diversity, and aware of complex and competing forces that influence women's relationships to systems of health care. A deep appreciation for the social worlds of women suffuses many of these books—including a valuing of women's relationships to their bodies, and their struggles for access to health care and new reproductive technologies. Recent writings on lesbian health—in particular—exhibit a powerful understanding of the politics of health care and the ways in which systems of oppression function to catalog bodies, rank their value, and regulate their social control.

Perhaps this distinction between writings on gay men's and lesbians' health is rooted in differently gendered relationships to community organizing and politics. As we end the century, there is a nascent, growing lesbian health movement in the United States, composed of health providers, activists, researchers, and theorists in dialogue with one another on topics that include cancer, depression, multiple sclerosis, diabetes, eating disorders, and violence. A number of lesbian cancer projects have formed, women's health programs have opened in a number of community-based clinics, and the Institute of Medicine has issued a major report on the state of lesbian health care, research, and treatment. Writings on lesbian health seem more deeply informed by feminism, social theory, and a social justice agenda, and collective action takes precedence over individual acts.

Gay men—like most men—are able to access health care more readily than our female counterparts, and are much more likely than lesbians to find health providers sensitive to our needs. Gay and lesbian health clinics continue to devote the vast majority of their resources to the needs of gay men, yet an important distinction needs to be made between receiving health services and participating in a health movement. While urban gay men are able to avail ourselves of gay-targeted services including STD screening and treatment, addiction recovery programs, smoking cessation support groups, and domestic violence counseling, we are not organized in anything resembling a comprehensive health care movement.

Lesbians energetically organize a health movement to expand resources, services, and research focused on lesbians, while contemporary gay men gaze out over the ruins of an AIDS movement struggling to remain alive yet refusing to reinvent itself in the wake of the major medical and cultural changes of the past decade. Beyond AIDS, gay men's health care needs are organized in a panoply of narrow categories—mental health, antiviolence, sexually transmitted diseases, substance abuse—and are rarely considered collectively from a holistic framework. When work occurs on gay men's health issues, superficial, individualistic solutions are offered and depoliticized analyses are put forward. Routinely, we are told gay men go to the gym because they have low self-esteem; young queer men fuck without condoms because they believe they're invulnerable; gay men use crystal meth because of internalized homophobia.

Thirty years after Stonewall, and twenty years after our victorious efforts to transform the American Psychiatric Association's stance on homosexuality, most writings on gay men's health continue to treat gay men as public health outlaws.

This is why Michael Scarce's work stands as an oasis amid an arid wasteland of writings on gay men's health. Whether writing about gay bowel syndrome, anal Pap smears, rectal microbicides, or the onset of the age of Viagra, Scarce understands that identities, bodies, and communities are complex sites in which to grapple with disease and wellness. By working simultaneously as a scholar, cultural critic, community activist, and emerging gay health expert, Scarce skillfully avoids the disciplinary wars that have wreaked havoc on the health sciences and brings a broad and rich perspective to his analysis. Scarce knows that the past thirty years of social theory offer rich possibilities for reconstructing gay male health activism and does not hesitate to draw on Judith Butler, Bruno Latour, and Anne Fausto-Sterling to inform and deepen his analysis. At the same time, his astute readings of contemporary texts and his ability to reimagine Miss America as a sexual disciplinarian, will ensure that this book reaches a wide audience.

It does not surprise me that the most insightful work on gay men's health in two decades comes from a twenty-eight-year-old gay man. Scarce is one of an emerging group of gay men who came out after the arrival of AIDS and who are rethinking gay identities and cultures. Along with gay men's health organizer Chris Bartlett of Philadelphia, sex advocate and writer Tony Valenzuela, journalist Wayne Hoffman, and health activist Ephen Colter, Scarce is part of the new generation of savvy queer organizers who approach gay men's health in new and exciting ways—with vision and without apology. Challenging the reigning AIDS-era "disciplinism" that makes use of a few narrow academic fields (behavioral psychology and epidemiology), this post-Foucaultian generation is revisiting our familiar, comfortable understandings of gay men's health and igniting a radical transformation.

Key to this new generation is a powerful critique of scientific knowledge that draws on the earlier AIDS-focused work of Jennifer Terry, Cindy Patton, and Steven Epstein to not only bridge culture and science, but actually view science for what it is: not a simple exposition of "facts," but a kind of cultural practice that—like every other culture practice—demands scrutiny and meticulous deconstruction. In this book, Scarce dives unabashedly into sociology of knowledge debates and creates important opportunities to influence, change, and ultimately democratize scientific research and practice.

While some may argue that Scarce's age and education level disqualify him from this task (he has just begun a PhD in medical sociology), it is precisely because of his ability to offer an outside critique that his work is fresh, innovative, and necessary. Democratization of medical science implies that useful critiques are likely to emerge from persons outside the field, just as one need not be a political scientist or a politician to critique life within Washington's beltway. The implications of placing the speculum into the hands of gay men again—taking back our bodies and our butts from the researchers and epidemiologists and gazing at them ourselves—may be profound.

Michael Scarce is the future of gay men's health, not because he has all the answers, but because he asks all the right questions and singlehandedly succeeds at moving forward with at least two major levels of contemporary discourse about our bodies and lives. With one foot firmly planted in cultural studies of science and the other in the feminist antiviolence movement, Scarce's work will hold only increasing relevance and importance in coming years as the AIDS glacier begins to melt and split up and other health issues seize prominent positions on the gay health agenda.

Smearing the Queer: Medical Bias in the Health Care of Gay Men is the book for which many of us have waited. By offering new theoretical frames for our work, and focusing his cultural and political critique on key critical health issues we face, Michael Scarce surely establishes himself as a leading voice catalyzing the gay men's health movement.

*   *   *

Eric Rofes is a long-time community organizer and the author of ten books, including *Dry Bones Breathe: Gay Men Creating Post-AIDS Identities and Culture* (The Haworth Press, 1998). He received his doctorate from UC Berkeley in social and cultural studies in education, and is Assistant Professor of Education at Humboldt State University, Arcata, California.

Acknowledgments

I am indebted to a number of people who helped make this book possible, including friends, colleagues, and acquaintances, as well as other writers and artists whose work has inspired me. Valuable feedback was provided by Jennifer Terry, Willa Young, Dottie Painter, Debra Moddelmog, David Horn, Matthew Brown, Ann Fausto-Sterling, William Byne, Eric Rofes, Verta Taylor, and Clark Taylor on various chapters that comprise this book. Folks at The Haworth Press, including Melissa Devendorf, Andy Roy, Sandy Jones Sickels, Bill Palmer, and John DeCecco, helped get these words into print.

In addition, friends and colleagues who provided much-needed encouragement and support throughout the writing and editing process include Marc Conte, Paul Morris, Marj Plumb, Tony Valenzuela, and others. Special thanks to Brian Oleksak, who was sweet enough to be supportive and understanding every time I said, "I need to write tonight."

A number of individuals' organizational work informed the structure and theory of this book, including Chris Bartlett and the work of Safe Guards in Philadelphia; Stephen Gibson and Stop AIDS Project of San Francisco; Project SIGMA in the United Kingdom; Eric Hildebrandt and Gay City in Seattle; Student Gender and Sexuality Services at Ohio State University; and Walter Armstrong and the staff of *POZ* magazine.

Kathy Fagan, David Citino, and fellow students in Ohio State University's English Department helped improve and challenge the poetry in this volume. Several of the poems were previously published elsewhere, including "A Recipe for Rectal Tarts" in *Diseased Pariah News,* "The Plumber's Applause" in *Mediphors: A Literary Journal of the Health Professions,* "Threadbare Back" in *Bay Windows,* and "Immaculate Infection" in University of Cincinnati's *Journal of Creative Social Discourse.*

As for visual accompaniments, Mary Ann Leeper of the Female Health Company was brave enough to grant permission to reprint the "investigative use only" instructions for rectal Reality. *Bon appétit* to artist Kira Od, who provided the hedonistic illustration accompanying my "Recipe for Rectal Tarts." Lastly, I am indebted to Linda Howard for creating the wonderful cover art, giving shape and form to the abstraction of my work.

Introduction

Fucking with Technology

> Biologists . . . write texts about human development. These documents, which take the form of research papers, texts, review articles, and popular books, grow from interpretations of scientific data. Because they represent scientific findings, one might imagine that they contain no preconceptions, no culturally instigated belief systems. But this turns out not to be the case. Although based on evidence, scientific writing can be seen as a particular kind of cultural interpretation—the enculturated scientist interprets nature. In the process, he or she also uses that interpretation to reinforce old or build new sets of social beliefs.[1]

Herein I have pulled together a critical, cultural analysis of contentious aspects of gay men's sexual health. The topics to which these chapters are devoted remain relatively unexamined outside the context of medical publications and infrequent mentionings in some popular media. My intent is to draw attention to a number of these issues, not only because of their possible benefit or harm to gay men, but to challenge the widespread neglect in pursuing their scientific, political, and cultural importance. While certainly these essays do not represent a comprehensive snapshot of contemporary concerns in gay male health and wellness, they do serve as points of illustration and exploration into the variety of ways in which social prejudices remain embedded in the health sciences. The complexity of power relations that structure health sciences today, ranging from shifting economic markets to clinical research imperatives, continue to mediate individuals' lives based on their affinity and participation in specific cultural groupings. In the case of sexuality, gay men reside among a number of social deviants with a problematic relationship to the fields of medicine, epidemiology, public health, pharmacology, psychiatry, and other health sciences. Mired in a historical model of homosexuality as pathology, one even begins to wonder exactly what a healthy gay man might look like.

The vast majority of thought and writing on gay male health since the early 1980s has concentrated, for some good reasons, on HIV and AIDS. Quite understandably, the decimation wrought by the epidemic and the political struggles bound up with community survival in the face of AIDS necessitated a focus on safer sex and care for those who were infected. Over time, however, this focus has resulted in a disturbingly narrow view of gay male sexual health, one predominantly limited to latex condoms and the treatment of complications resulting from a single virus. Until quite recently, AIDS had become the prevailing metaphor for gay men's health. Education and prevention efforts revolving around other sexually transmitted infections, substance abuse, violence, mental health, and a myriad of other concerns took a back seat to the AIDS epidemic in most urban gay communities.

By the late 1990s, a resurgence in the attention to comprehensive gay male health began to emerge as many gay men no longer experienced AIDS as a crisis. This makes sense given that the very definition of a crisis is a temporary situation that ends in some form of resolution. The epidemic continues, of course, but writers and scholars like Eric Rofes have documented a shift from crisis mentality to negotiated resolution as gay men struggle to find meaning and community over the long haul.[2] At the same time, scientific advances have yielded a host of new technologies, many of which possess the potential to revolutionize sexual behaviors and the meanings associated with them. When applied to gay male bodies, these technologies create opportunities to dramatically enable or substantially impede not only quality of health, but sexual pleasure, political progress, cultural advancement, and community empowerment. This book represents an attempt to begin a critical examination of these technologies both within and outside the context of AIDS, interrogating how health scientists use these tools to classify and characterize differing forms of sexuality, why some gay men appropriate these technologies for unintended and often unapproved use, the criteria by which access to these technologies is granted or restricted, and more broadly, how new applications of health science will continue to dramatically shape gay men's lives over time.

The title of this volume, *Smearing the Queer*, represents not only a childhood game based on a premise of antigay violence, but a larger ideology that positions gay male sexuality as something to be violated in a punitive fashion, instructive in its message communicated and lesson learned. In addition, the smeared queer is situated on a border of sex and disease, embodied by a resistance to taxonomy, and elusive in a fluidity of performances, identities, and representations. The persistence of homophobia and heterosexism throughout facets of health science converge at the two primary points of treatment and research as vehicles for smearing the queer both literally and figuratively. Through an emphasis on the body and its constituent parts, health sciences work as a cultural practice to construct queer bodies and the social forces that govern them, while at the same time being confounded by a queer resistance that transgresses scientific claims to order and authority.

The essays and poems comprising this collection of scientifically smeared queers are divided into three sections, each representing a different definition of the word smear. Section I, dedicated to the meaning of smear as a form of slander, includes an article on gay bowel syndrome that was published in an earlier form in the *Journal of Homosexuality*. For years, scholars and activists have discussed AIDS, first dubbed gay-related immune deficiency (GRID), as the first official gay disease. Gay bowel syndrome predates AIDS by several years, however, offering contradiction even to the medical notion of the "previously healthy homosexual" so prevalent in early AIDS discourse. Whereas the term GRID was abandoned rather quickly after it was coined, gay bowel syndrome has survived for more than twenty years and continues to be used as medical evidence against gay men in political struggles ranging from employment discrimination to adoption rights.

Section II encompasses smearing as the action of spreading a wet substance across a surface. The two chapters comprising this section examine new safer sex technologies, their impact on gay men, and the politics of their appropriation. Gay men's use of so-called "female-controlled" products such as the Reality Female Condom for anal intercourse draws attention to the increasingly problematic restriction of access to new safer sex measures. This is compounded by the fact that, almost two decades into the AIDS pandemic, the United States government still has not approved a single condom or other barrier for anal sex. The almost exclusive focus on vaginal protection in the scientific research agenda for future development of microbicides as a kind of chemical prophylaxis is equally disturbing. Crossing lines of gender as well as sexuality, the engagement of users with devices for sexual purposes has troubled the notions of scientific enablement, public health strategies for disease prevention, and the federal government's role in regulating products for a sexual marketplace.

Section III refers to the smear as a prepared medium for microscopic examination. The heightened scrutiny of gay male bodies, coupled with increasingly sophisticated screening technologies, has created new opportunities for monitoring potential disease as well as inscribing gay male bodies within a renewed context of perversion and sexual pathology. In the case of anal cancer in gay men, the Pap smear is a prospective tool for early detection and intervention of disease, yet federal agencies and medical professional organizations have refused to develop or adopt a protocol for effective screening. Together, the chapters on the Reality female condom, microbicides for sexual acts, and Pap smear procedures make a clear case for why the health of women and gay men have become inextricably linked through health sciences and technologies, demanding closer alliance and collaboration between social movements vested with these interests. Also included in this section is a chapter titled "Something Borrowed, Something Blue" fleshing out some work I presented as a panelist during a San Francisco town hall meeting on gay men's use of Viagra.

The concluding section, "Clearing the Smear," includes a fictional medical journal article titled "Heterocopulative Syndrome." The piece was written as a form of oppositional narrative, intended to reveal a number of the inherent contradictions and biases built into purportedly objective medical science. Although somewhat tongue in cheek, the mimicry of medical journal text as a kind of genre literature unto itself is helpful for examining heterosexist methodology and interpretation throughout the field.

The collected text of these essays may present two troubling qualities for some readers. First, the tone of the chapters varies slightly; some are written in academic prose, while others are of a more popular style, and even poems have been interspersed as commentary on related content. Differences in the kinds of analyses, sources of original publication in earlier forms, and topics of the pieces have all influenced my decision to write this book as a somewhat interdisciplinary assemblage. Second, the contemporary nature of many themes addressed herein create the distinct possibility that some of the information will become dated in a relatively short period of time. Such is the nature of writing on matters such as rapidly changing technologies, unfortunately. Documentation of gay men's relationship to health sciences at this juncture is valuable nonetheless.

As a whole, the book enumerates thematic strategies for improving relations between gay men and the health sciences by building a broader-based agenda for gay health advocacy, challenging heterosexist bias within health care delivery and health sciences research, and calling for the development of public policy initiatives to provide frameworks for addressing gay men's wellness in more sophisticated and complex ways.

SECTION I:
SMEAR AS DEFAMATION

Dr. Kazal's Ace in the Hole

There once was a doc named Kazal
whose research was rather banal
until when one day,
he named a bowel "Gay"
and taught it a language quite foul.

This bowel soon became quite a puppet.
Using his hand, he would stuff it.
It became such a game
of stigma and shame
that no ace in this hole could trump it.

The signs and the symptoms were there.
They needed sound medical care.
Gay bowels had no choice,
were given a voice,
and translated into a scare.

Kazal had medical expertise,
interpreting things he would grease.
Pieces were assembled
until they resembled
a language of syndromic disease.

This language is quite easily spoken
by body parts fragmented and broken.
Urban bums now moan
of lost muscle tone
and rough rides costing more than coined tokens.

Chapter 1

Harbinger of Plague:
A Bad Case of Gay Bowel Syndrome

I first discovered the term "gay bowel syndrome" in 1994, buried in a medical journal article on emergency room treatment of adult male rape survivors. Working as an AIDS educator a few months later, I received in the mail a sample educational brochure on sexually transmitted diseases that included a short description of gay bowel syndrome. The appearance of this gay disease in clinical research and public health campaign texts intrigued me, both in the manner in which the notion of a gay disease seemed to be treated as publicly acceptable and medically factual, as well as the durability of such a term across the span of several years. The queer activist in me was angered by what I judged to be blatant medical homophobia, while the queer scholar in me became deeply interested in the construction of scientific fact in application of the syndrome to gay male bodies.

A great deal is at stake in viewing scientific knowledge as culturally constructed knowledge, for this allows one to begin to understand science within its context, not simply as unquestionable truth and objective fact. To say that scientific facts are culturally constructed is to point to a degree of cultural consensus. A concept becomes a fact through an agreement to define an idea, theory, or explanation as such.[1] A study of scientific knowledge can reveal as much about the culture from which it was produced as the world which it attempts to explain and unravel. Analysis of the process of fact building through a consensus between individuals, communities, and systems can make clear the establishment of authority and stability granted to scientific knowledge in its cultural context. The reflexive acknowledgment that sciences are laden with the values of the cultures from which they stem provides an entrypoint for disruption in the sense of reimagining scientific knowledge in ways that are less sexist, racist, classist, and heterosexist.

Through medical journal discourse as a cultural production of scientific facts, physicians and researchers have been able to construct, fragment, and reconstruct human bodies in highly narrativized and politically charged ways. Often these bodies are depicted as deviant by means of literal and figurative dissection, an excision and objectification of body parts for characterization and cultural coding. In understandings of disease as a construction of culture, the influence of medical discourse becomes key in the connoting and legitimating of bodily representations. Through this process of cultural production, the fragmentation of bodies into broken and disordered parts often creates an identity based upon and conceptualized through models of disease.

In their introduction to *Deviant Bodies*, an anthology seeking to map embodied deviance, editors Jennifer Terry and Jacqueline Urla write, "The somatic territorializing of deviance, since the nineteenth century, has been part and parcel of a larger effort to organize social relations according to categories denoting normality versus aberration, health versus pathology, and national security versus social danger."[2] The policing of bodies found to be socially deviant has often been undertaken in the name of public health and grounded in the authority of medical science. Health becomes equated with morality and measures are often taken by policy makers to necessitate the restriction of a population's liberties in support of the ever-vulnerable, common good of the moral majority.

In his article, "Moral Contagion and the Medicalizing of Gay Identity: AIDS in Historical Perspective," Steven Epstein identifies the 1970s venereal disease specialists' view of sexually transmitted diseases as intrinsic to the modern, urban, male homosexual subculture.[3] He suggests this view of sexually diseased (both physiologically and sociologically) gay men subsequently facilitated the 1980s construction of AIDS as a gay disease and homosexuality, therefore, as a contemporary moral and medical menace.[4] The historical links between sexually transmitted diseases (STDs) found in urban gay communities in the 1970s and their later connections to AIDS and homosexuality have remained rather ambiguous, however. In what ways did popular and scientific perceptions of these STDs and gay men lay the groundwork for medical science's identification of gay men as an epidemiologically significant population? Similarly, how did these perceptions reconfigure social constructions of gay men as morally contagious and socially dangerous?

I have attempted here to sketch a picture of the construction, definition, development, and application of an identified collection of sexually transmitted diseases and proctologic (related to the anus, rectum, or colon) conditions that, together, have been defined by medical researchers as constituting the "gay bowel syndrome." Based on Epstein's premise that such pre-AIDS discourses as gay bowel syndrome set the stage for a relatively easy process of scapegoating gay men and the homophobic construction and implementation of AIDS as a gay disease, I wish to investigate these connections between gay bowel syndrome and AIDS. This will also assist with my inquiry into the ways in which gay bowel syndrome has been, and remains today, a powerful tool for the specific surveillance, regulation, definition, medicalization, identification, and fragmentation of gay men's bodies.

The history of the smear campaign of gay bowel syndrome which I have pieced together is by no means exhaustive, but I aim to create a clear enough picture to indicate gay bowel syndrome's significance to gay identity, medical science, and relations of power spanning the past twenty years. I have drawn upon a range of cultural sources to do this work, primarily textual, that include medical journals and other scientific texts; sexually transmitted disease educational pamphlets and literature; newspaper, magazine, and wire report articles; instructional sex manuals; and transcripts from such arenas as legislative testimony before Congress, medical conference proceedings, and national television news programs.

I have adopted methods from the works of Paula Treichler, Cindy Patton, and Steven Epstein in my examination of biomedical discourse and its impact upon our understandings of human bodies. Paula Treichler, for example, advises us to be critical in our approach to the reading of science as a cultural production, for "scientific and medical discourses have traditions through which the semantic epidemic as well as the biological one is controlled, and these may disguise contradiction and irrationality."[5] Resisting the discourse that masquerades as compelling certainty that Treichler and others write about is no easy task, however, for such discourse carries an arsenal of dismissals, self-exemptions, and alibis to thwart the would-be critic of medicine.

With this critical analysis in mind, I now turn to gay bowel syndrome's debut, which occurred in 1976 within the pages of the *Annals of Clinical and Laboratory Science.*[6] The article, "The Gay Bowel Syndrome: Clinico-Pathologic Correlation in 260 Cases," by Henry L. Kazal and his four co-authors, documents a pattern of sexually transmitted anorectal and colonic diseases encountered in 260 predominantly white, middle- to upper-class, gay men who had visited a private proctologic practice in New York City. The authors christened their patients' pattern of multiple proctologic afflictions as gay bowel syndrome, "a group of anorectal and colon conditions found with unusual frequency in male homosexuals."[7] Clinical diagnoses of these patients included twenty-two conditions (in descending order of prevalence): condyloma acuminata (genital warts), hemorrhoids, nonspecific proctitis, anal fistula, perirectal abscess, anal fissure, amebiasis, pruritus ani, polyps (benign), hepatitis, rectal dyspareunia, gonorrhea, syphilis, trauma and foreign bodies, shigellosis, rectal ulcers, lymphogranuloma venereum, anal incontinence, solitary rectal ulcer, Bowen's disease, squamous cell carcinoma, and an "other" classification. The frequency of these conditions is never quantified nor contextualized as unusual in comparison to other epidemiological studies. The definition of gay bowel syndrome, from its inception, is unclear.

Only demographic breakdowns of age and occupation of the men were offered in the article. Biopsy results of 51 of the 260 men are discussed in more depth. Based on the researchers' findings, the article encourages physicians to broaden the scope of their medical examinations and diagnoses to encompass more than the five traditional venereal diseases of that time when dealing with homosexual male patients: syphilis, gonorrhea, herpes, condyloma, and chlamydia.

Three specific case studies are given in greater detail: a twenty-year-old white male student, a forty-three-year-old white male professor, and a thirty-eight-year-old white male television producer. Kazal and his fellow researchers fail to state with any determination exactly how they define gay, or how they have identified these men as such. They do state that a complete sexual history was not obtained from all the patients. Clearly, these physicians were not certain their patients even identified as gay, or had necessarily engaged in same-sex sexual practices, as evidenced by statements such as, "In the absence of a history of homosexuality, the physician may be alerted to the gay bowel syndrome by anal condyloma acuminata (anal warts). When this sentinel lesion is not present, the syndrome may be suspected by a constellation of other findings."[8] The troubling category of gay is invoked, but a definition is carefully avoided.

One year later in 1977, a similar article was published in the *American Journal of Gastroenterology* by Norman Sohn and James Robilotti, both of whom had co-authored the original Kazal and colleagues piece. Their article, however, possesses some notably different characteristics. First, the term gay bowel syndrome from the Kazal article became capitalized in the Sohn and Robilotti article as Gay Bowel Syndrome. The capitalization, while a minor change, does in some ways represent the progression of the term as it incrementally accumulated authority and importance. This was no longer simply a detected pattern of disease, but had become an Official Illness. In addition, it is curious that the Sohn and Robilotti article does not cite or mention the Kazal and colleagues article that had been published one year previously. One would suspect that if these researchers were attempting to build a body of gay bowel syndrome literature, cross-references and citations to other pieces of research on the syndrome would be of significance. Sohn and Robilotti also distinguish gay bowel syndrome as an emerging, newly recognized collection of polymicrobial, sexually transmitted "diseases not heretofore associated with any particular sexual activity."[9] They also add to the original Kazal study the descriptor of gay bowel syndrome conditions being "recurrent."

The Sohn and Robilotti article is a duplication of the first Kazal and colleagues article in many ways. They discuss the same 260 gay male patients in the same private practice in New York City, naming almost identical characteristics of the syndrome. They do, however, offer a working definition of homosexual (in describing an act, not an identity) that the 1976 article did not provide:

> For the purpose of this report, we are defining male homosexual behavior as any sexual relationship, including orogenital, proctogenital, or analingual sex between two or more males. The fact that the patient has had or is now having heterosexual relationships is irrelevant to the topic of discussion. Previous male homosexual activity, even if represented by a single experience, exposes the patient to the conditions under consideration.[10]

A same-sex sexual encounter is framed here in terms of exposure to the diseases and conditions that constitute gay bowel syndrome. Five of the 260 patients in the study were married to women, but they are considered homosexual as well. Throughout the article, references to homosexual behavior interchange with homosexual men, as the deviant behavior of same-sex sexuality takes precedence as a descriptive label for the patients over any heterosexual self-identification or practices. Concern for the health of these men's female sexual partners who might also have been placed at risk for these transmittable conditions is also ignored.

The third appearance of gay bowel syndrome in a medical journal occurred three years later in 1980 with "The Gay Bowel Syndrome: A Common Problem of Homosexual Patients in the Emergency Department" by Dr. Michael Heller, director of the Division of Emergency Medicine at University of California, San Francisco's Moffitt Hospital. This is the first evidence of the term being used on the west coast, and the article published in the *Annals of Emergency Medicine* gave gay bowel syndrome a sense of urgency and dire consequence. Gay bowel syndrome was not just a complication needing treatment in a quiet private practice, but could become severe enough to necessitate crisis and trauma intervention. Heller uses this urgency in his encouragement of physicians learning more about gay bowel syndrome: "Most physicians are simply not aware of the spectrum of sexually transmitted bowel disease in gays. The syndrome has not been widely reported outside specialty journals and has not yet been included in standard texts."[11]

Ten more journal articles focusing on homosexual men's rectal health followed throughout the 1980s authoritatively invoking and diagnosing gay bowel syndrome as an official medical term via citation of these first three articles.[12] Gay bowel syndrome's place was thus secured in the canonized nomenclature of disease as first conceptualized by this handful of physicians specializing in proctologic and emergency medicine. These researchers made no revolutionary discovery in their detection of a pattern among gay male patients. Rather, they formulated connections between 1970s sexual liberation, rising STD rates, and the promiscuity of some gay men by creating a syndrome to embody and typify these connections.

More than fifteen journal articles and other medical science texts published after Kazal et al., in chronological succession, have expanded and diversified the possible constituent components of gay bowel syndrome to a practically all-encompassing degree, rendering the term gay bowel syndrome virtually meaningless in its breadth of scope. Gay bowel syndrome began as a semidefinitive collection consisting of twenty-two variations of bacteria, virus, parasites, and a small hodgepodge of miscellaneous proctologic complications (such as inflammations, cancers, trauma, and more). Within a decade, other medical authorities had added their own compositional elements to gay bowel syndrome until the laundry list of conditions had exceeded well over fifty items. (See Table 1.1.)

I have described in more depth the first three appearances of gay bowel syndrome in 1976, 1977, and 1980 for a specific reason: they all predate the widespread recognition of AIDS and the heightened medical scrutiny of gay men that would shortly follow. For five years, gay bowel syndrome was relegated to medical specialty journals and a scarce mentioning in the gay press. By late 1981 and early 1982, however, a great deal of attention was directed to the topic of gay disease as more and more gay men were found to have debilitating immune system deficiencies. Discussions, mentionings, and references to gay bowel syndrome increased dramatically after 1981, as did the arena of gay bowel syndrome discourse. Gay bowel syndrome would soon make its popular appearance in the pages of *Time* magazine, major newspapers, and national television as a highly politicized and hotly contested construct.

TABLE 1.1. Conditions Included in the Composition of Gay Bowel Syndrome

Virus

Condyloma acuminatum
Cytomegalovirus
Hepatitis A
Hepatitis B
Hepatitis C
Herpes I
Herpes II
Human herpes virus 8 (HHV-8)
Human immunodeficiency virus (HIV)

Bacteria

Brachyspira aalborgii (intestinal spirochetosis)
Branhamella catarrhalis
Calymmatobacterium granulomatis
Campylobacter fetus (formerly named Vibrio fetus)
Chlamydia trachomatis
Enterotoxogenic escherichia coli (E. coli)
Gonorrhea
Hemophilus ducreyi
Mycobacterium avium intracellulare
Neisseria meningitidis
Nongonococcal urethritis
Salmonella
Shigella
Syphilis
Treponema pallidum

Parasites

Blastocystis haminis
Cryptosporidia
Dientamoeba fragilis
Entamoeba coli
Entamoeba hartmanni
Entamoeba histolytica
Entamoeba nana
Enterobius vermincularis
Giardiasis (Giardia lamblia)
Iodamoeba butschlii
Isospora belli
Microsporidiosis
"Non-pathonogenic" parasites
Pneumocystis carinii (enteric)
Pneumocystis carinii pneumonia

Other Parasites (*continued*)

Strongyloidiasis
"Worms of many varieties"

Other

Allergic proctitis (from medicinal creams or foams)
Anal fissure
Anal fistula
Anal incontinence
Bowen's disease, anus
Enteritis
Foreign body (includes fisting)
Hemorrhoid
"HIV enteropathy"
Intestinal perforation
Kaposi's sarcoma
Laceration
Lymphopathy
Non-specific proctitis
Penile edema
Perineal sepsis
Perirectal abscess
Polyps (benign)
Proctocolitis
Pruritus ani
Rectal dyspareunia
Rectal tears
Rectal ulcer
Sexual assault
Squamous cell carcinoma

GAYING THE BOWEL

Apart from the lack of a standardized and concrete working definition of gay bowel syndrome, the nomenclature of such a malady is additionally problematic. The gayness of gay bowel syndrome is of particular concern in this allegory of culpability. Surprisingly, particular usage of the word gay rather than homosexual in medical literature was rare for 1976, although the two are used interchangeably throughout the gay bowel syndrome journal articles. None of the researchers offers a definition of gay, and it remains a fluid term in the literature, sometimes used to connote a history of sexual acts, sometimes identity, and often both.

First, one must consider what exactly makes this bowel syndrome gay. Specifying the bowel as a gay bowel marks the homosexual male body as being somehow physically different, unique in its diseased physiology as a result of perverse practices. This serves to erase the conceptual possibility of heterosexual anal activity while establishing a sense of safety in a distance from the illness and dangerous contagion of the homo-other. However, not all gay men's sexual practices involve anal activity, and not all gay men are even sexually active. Many heterosexual people and lesbian women find pleasure in anal activities. Rather easily, the contradictions in a gay syndrome are offered by those who continue its characterization and utility, found in such awkward disclaimers as:

- Sexual transmission of enteric diseases is neither new nor limited to gays.[13]
- In evaluating proctologic problems in gay males, it is apparent that all of the sexually transmitted microorganisms that infect the heterosexual population should be considered.[14]
- These disorders are by no means exclusive to this population, but epidemiologically they appear more frequently.[15]
- Gay bowel syndrome is a misnomer in that homosexuality is not a risk factor for development of the syndrome.[16]
- It is apparent that homosexuals are not uniquely at risk for venereal transmission of enteric organisms. Heterosexual anal intercourse or analingus may transmit infection if one of the partners harbors a pathogen.[17]

If gay bowel syndrome was considered by these physicians to be a misnomer or in some way inaccurate, why do they perpetuate its continuation by using it in their publications to refer to sexually transmitted diseases?

If heterosexual people have also been diagnosed with the conditions that constitute gay bowel syndrome, if heterosexual anal acts can (and do) transmit or inflict such conditions, and if not all gay men participate in anal sexual practices, then the only remaining scientific and political justification for a gay disease relies upon the epidemiological prevalence of such conditions found largely in a particular social and geographic population. This, of course, is not only a generalization, but the kind of glaring bias of which objective science purports to be devoid, for there have emerged no new diseases such as straight male urethral syndrome nor a heterocopulant vagina disorder. While diseases such as pelvic inflammatory disease may be attributed only to heterosexual women, for instance, the name of the disease is not constricted to a designated epidemiological population. There is no presumption of a community site for heterosexual disease. This distinguishes gay bowel syndrome, in both its attribution and characterization, as a somewhat unique form of representation of subordinated bodies. While other illnesses have been named after socially constructed categorizations of people, such as Legionnaire's disease, they have typically not borne such an air of blame-the-victim persecution.

So what functions, then, do the gaying of anal pleasure, anal practices, and their perceived negative consequences serve? The designation of the descriptive gay marks not only an imagined typology of sexual practice but a gender coding. If gay also indicates male, certain heterosexual panics might be soothed since the anus eludes a stable gender categorization. Cindy Patton discusses the heterodenial of anal pleasure and desire as the function of a logic that "constructs a double safety: they do not practice this risk behavior nor do they possess the queer desires that lead to it."[18] The use of gay bowel syndrome as a tool for categorizing difference reinforces this construction of safety, for it forecloses heterosexual anxieties of disease and the consensual relinquishing of heterosexual masculinity via penetration of the male anus. This is not to say, however, that heterosexuality is always deemed normal and moral, nor that heterosexual practices can be deviant only if they are related to the rectum.[19]

Simon Watney writes of an anxiety-ridden social necessity of the homosexual body, whose ideological function "exposes the more or less desperate ambition to confine mobile desire in the semblance of a stable object, calibrated by its sexual aim, regarded as a 'wrong choice.' The 'homosexual body' would thus evidence a fictive collectivity of perverse sexual performances, denied any psychical reality and pushed out beyond the farthest margins of the social."[20] In application of Watney's understanding of the homosexual body, one can see how gay bowel syndrome is easily configured in a constellatory arrangement as a representation of the gay male body, symbolizing its inherent pathology, marking its perverse nature and menace to society for all to behold.

Since the definition of gay bowel syndrome includes physical trauma to the anus or rectum, anal rape and sexual assault become qualifying conditions as well. One of the gay bowel syndrome complications listed by Silfen and Stair are "rectal tears resulting from rape or insertion of foreign object or hand."[21] Medically speaking, being anally raped may classify a man as gay via a diagnosis of gay bowel syndrome. This perpetuates the popular misconception that sexually assaulting a person of the same sex will "make them gay."

In a case study of a patient presenting with rectal trauma as the result of being anally gang-raped, Chen, Davis, and Ott diagnose the rape survivor as having gay bowel syndrome.[22] The diagnosis is made in the absence of any apparent parasitic or other infectious agent, and is simply due to tissue damage from an injury inflicted through violence. The sexual identity of the rape survivor is never stated, although it is certainly implied. The gay diagnostic label serves as an excellent example of cultural confusion between sex and violence.

Same-sex rape becomes equated with same-sex, consensual sexual activity, conjuring images of the predatory homosexual as molester of children and opportunistic perpetrator.[23] In this way, all anal sex becomes assaultive as an unhealthy behavior. Penetration is equated with violation. Heterosexual men are advised by society, "Don't drop the soap" in the presence of the male homosexual—for the heterosexual man who makes himself vulnerable to anal penetration will become stricken with the affliction (homosexuality) of his homosexual rapist.

This anxiety is symptomatic of the particular dangers found in gay bowel syndrome, that it is a malady which is acquired rather than inherited. In her sketching of a brief history of the scientific search for homosexual bodies, Jennifer Terry poses the question, "If homosexuality is signified through the body, are its marks the *source* or the *consequence* of experiences and desires?"[24] The answer is often both. Body significations of homosexuality are sometimes constructed to be the source of experiences and desires, while sometimes they are the consequence. The body is then marked in ways that medical authorities purport to read or interpret (i.e., diagnose) based on expert opinion. Gay bowel syndrome serves as an example of a signifier acquired through participation (consensually or otherwise) in socially deviant acts, although an underlying predisposition toward it seems to be at work as well.

SITING THE BOWEL

Of additional concern is the bowel in gay bowel syndrome. Several of the noted conditions of gay bowel syndrome involve exterior (perianal) skin, such as herpes, genital warts, external hemorrhoids, and physical trauma. Contact with a mouth, penis, or anus is not required for transmission or infliction of such external complications, for skin-to-skin contact may be sufficient, as in the case of herpes and variations of human papilloma virus (warts). In addition, gay bowel syndrome names only the "receptacle," the site or receiving end of infection or complication. None of the conditions constituting gay bowel syndrome is transmitted or inflicted directly *from* bowel *to* bowel. Rather, an infected penis, mouth, finger, or other transporter must deliver a pathogen from its source to the anus, rectum, or colon either directly or through ingestion.

So why is gay bowel syndrome localized to the bowel? Perhaps the perceptions of uncleanliness, coupled with deviant unnaturalness of the bowel as a site of pleasure, incriminate this anatomical locale as a likely landscape of disease. Misogyny in the form of feminine passivity (defined by medical authorities as penetrability) is also indicated, for to be sexually penetrated is to court infectious danger. Kazal and colleagues attribute the high number of cases of gay bowel syndrome in their practice to a "preference in these patients for a receptor (female) role."[25] Gay men who practice receptive anal intercourse are equated with female bodies in no uncertain terms here, with the exception that the anus is more vulnerable than the vagina.[26] As Leo Bersani wrote fifteen years after the publication of the Kazal and colleagues article, "Women and gay men spread their legs with an unquenchable appetite for destruction."[27] Since no self-respecting heterosexual man should want to be anally penetrated, and since men who are raped "become" gay through medical diagnoses or confusion between rape and consensual sex, straight men are categorically devoid of the "fuck me" appetite and its subsequently wrought destruction.

Further, this scientific belief in the anus as a poorly chosen substitute for the vagina is quite prevalent, even amongst supposed pro-gay and gay medical practitioners. In a 1977 *Advocate* (a national gay news magazine) article, journalist Randy Shilts reported on an emerging plague of gastrointestinal diseases in gay men stemming from "the gymnastics of gay sex."[28] Shilts quoted Dan Williams, the medical director of New York's Gay Men's Health Project, as stating, "We're shy one orifice." Again, the implied missing orifice is the vagina—the natural, healthy, and normal site of sexual receptivity. Gay men become deficient and deviant in this respect. As traitors to traditional heterosexual masculinity, gay men pay the price for feminizing their bodies and allowing themselves to be penetrated.

The proctologic emphasis of siting gay bowel syndrome within the bowel might also be the relatively recent development of technologies that localizes disease to a specific part of the body while, at the same time, reveals its relationship to the rest of the body and other systems of anatomical function. New imaging technologies for parasitic detection and more sophisticated measures for testing bacteria and virus have enabled medical practitioners to tie highly localized pathogens to more general bodily symptoms such as fever, fatigue, nausea, respiratory difficulty, or diarrhea.

SPEAKING IN SYNDROMES

This consideration of homosexual bodily signification illuminates the final self-evident contradiction in gay bowel syndrome—the concept of the syndrome itself. One medical dictionary defines a syndrome to be "a group of symptoms and signs of disordered function related to one another by means of some anatomic, physiologic, or biochemical peculiarity."[29] This definition does not include a precise cause of illness, but does provide a framework of reference for investigating it. However, if a constellation effect of uncertain etiology is the major defining element of a syndrome, this too fails to be logical, because all the possible fifty-plus constitutive elements are of a fairly certain, known cause.

So where does the uncertainty that warrants a syndromic definition come into play? In the case of gay bowel syndrome, this syndromic peculiarity is a queer one, as the "anatomic, physiologic, or biochemical" homosexual male body is essentialized through scientific belief of same-sex sexuality to be of disordered function. In addition to the bowel, the syndrome in gay bowel syndrome reiterates the physicality of difference acquired through sexual practices while simultaneously hinting at an underlying, uncertain, essential difference that predisposes one to such an acquisition. The naming of these differences, collectively, varies from underlying processes to disease, to syndrome, as evidenced by the interchangeable uses of the terms gay bowel disease and gay bowel syndrome in medical texts and more popular cultural outlets. This constructed holism of gay bowel syndrome versus the fragmentation of gay bowel disease is mirrored by the anatomical specificity of the gay bowel and the larger systemic, essentialized homosexual body it operates within, producing an interaction between broken, damaged, fragmented body parts and an imaginary, inherently queer body.

Gay bowel syndrome is often defined as "multiple enteric infections [occurring] concurrently or sequentially,"[30] or a singular recurrent pathogen. Medical science tries to make sense of these pathogenic patterns through attempts at logically ordering them into systems of relationships called syndromes. Distinctions between diseases and syndromes are of incredible import, however, as Jan Zita Grover has shown in her article "AIDS: Keywords." She relates that "a syndrome points to or signifies the underlying disease process(es), while a disease is constituted by those processes. This is not merely a semantic distinction. Diseases can be communicable, syndromes cannot."[31] Acquired immune deficiency syndrome, for example, is not communicable, nor can the majority of opportunistic infections comprising the syndrome be transmitted to a person with a relatively healthy immune system. Rather, what is transmitted and acquired is human immunodeficiency virus. Gay bowel syndrome, on the other hand, is described by medical researchers as a constellation of conditions; but unlike AIDS, a communicable factor or some underlying phenomenon (such as

HIV) is never clearly stated or named—other than homosexuality as the nomenclature indicates.

In the case of AIDS, diseases (opportunistic infections) manifest as symptoms of an underlying HIV infection producing immune deficiency. With gay bowel syndrome, one or more of fifty-some diseases or conditions manifest as symptoms of an underlying pathology that is never clearly distinguished as specifically social or biological, which again brings us back to the question: gay bowel syndrome, as a marker of homosexuality signified through the body, is clearly constructed to be a consequence of homosexual practices, but is homosexuality the source of such bodily markers? Perhaps it is not the communicability/transmission (e.g., homosexual practices) of diseases comprising gay bowel syndrome that makes it a syndrome by medical definition, but, as Grover indicates, the underlying processes constituting such diseases. These unnamed "underlying processes" hint at some essentialized weaknesses, defective mechanisms, or predispositions in the constitution of the homosexual body that gives rise to the processes constituting the diseases.

These syndromes are not harmless models of abstract thought and reference, however. The medical domain's power of classification and nomenclature is constructed to be infinitely expandable in the definition of maladies that are specific to social and cultural groupings of human bodies. Speaking of gay bowel syndrome, one researcher notes, "There is no doubt that our traditional conceptions of sexually transmitted disease were too narrow; it is only slightly less certain that our current understanding of gay bowel disease will expand and develop as new etiologies are implicated and new clinical syndromes described."[32] Statements such as these reserve medical science's right to continuously update and revise the definitions of gay health and illness, while maintaining a space in which gay men can be perpetually objectified, fragmented, and scapegoated as responsible for any medical, and therefore social, problems that may arise. The language of syndromic constellation provides the alluring narrative needed to discursively weave the all-too-believable fable titled "Gay Bowel Syndrome." The openness of syndromic definition licensed an unfettered embellishment, and this tale of perversity and plague grew taller and taller.

DUAL DIAGNOSES

Physicians' diagnoses of gay bowel syndrome consist of two main processes that serve as instructive texts in their provision of step-by-step protocols for the management of such practices.[33] The two components of a gay bowel syndrome diagnosis are an attempted determination of the patient's sexual preference and the identification of any real, presumed, or possible proctologic conditions in the above mentioned fifty-plus item list. The two components of this diagnosis do not necessarily occur in this order. Male homosexual activity may lead to investigation of proctologic conditions, or vice versa, as each implicates the other in homophobic stereotype.

A history of homosexual behavior may be offered by the patient, or may simply be the presumption or suspicion of the physician. "There are certain physical findings which, while not absolutely diagnostic, should alert the examiner to the possibility of homosexuality."[34] Three of these four findings are the presence of anal warts, diminished anal sphincter tone, and a relaxation of the anal sphincter muscle. "The fourth sign can be termed the 'O' sign, in which the patient voluntarily is capable of maintaining the anus in a dilated position. This sign was present in approximately 4 percent of the patients."[35] Since these conditions of gay bowel syndrome might give voice to the rectum's confession of homosexual history, these telltale signs become a privileged part of the diagnostic inquisition. "The typical patient has a history of multiple diseases, which tend to recur. When alert to this clinical pattern, the physician may recognize the gay bowel syndrome even before a history of homosexuality has been elicited."[36] This homosexual identification becomes crucial, for not a single medical text citing gay bowel syndrome contains a case study or imagined possibility of a heterosexual person being diagnosed with the disease.

The homosexual male body is reconstructed here yet again, with specific bodily markers for not only the illness (gay bowel syndrome) but homosexuality itself, until the two become inseparable; for this is the Greek origin of the word syndrome—to run together.[37] This smearing in the smear campaign of gay bowel syndrome is not only one of reputation and blame, but of blurring any fragile boundaries between what constitutes the conceptual realms of disease and homosexuality. Pathology and homosexuality run together in a smudge of conflation which post-Stonewall gay organizing and activism has so vehemently sought to separate.

Gay bowel syndrome medical journal articles are implemented as proctologic mouthpieces, whispering the disclosure that same-sex sexual behaviors in and of themselves cause disease. "Frequency, number, and anonymity of sexual contacts among homosexual men, which are all facilitated at public baths and 'gay bars'" are given by Silfen and Stair as reasons for the emergence of new gay diseases, as is their perception of gay men as a "highly mobile population" and "'new' sexual practices such as analingus, which allow fecal-oral transmission of organisms."[38]

In addition, this body of literature suggests that same-sex sexual practices *are* diseases, complete with at least the four physical symptoms mentioned previously. Distinctions between act and actor are neatly collapsed into a densely performative homosexual male body, easily diagnosed in its vulnerably symptomatic state. Whereas Susan Sontag has pointed to the uses of illness as metaphor, through this slippery collapse, homosexuality and disease in this case no longer serve as metaphors for each other, for they have been culturally melded into synonymous indistinctness.

PREVENTION

If one considers for the sake of argument that gay bowel syndrome is a real syndrome, and not all gay men have gay bowel syndrome, then it must be avoidable or preventable. Kazal and colleagues observe that in 1970s' gay male sexual practices, "Chemical and mechanical prophylaxis is seldom used." [39] One year later, Sohn and Robilotti, who co-authored the original Kazal article, stated with certainty "There are no practical technics available for preventing the spread of venereal disease among male homosexuals aside from abstinence."[40]

A contradiction is made apparent in the comparison of these two notations. Gay men are deemed responsible for the spread of gay bowel syndrome, since they seldom enact chemical or mechanical preventive measures. The same authors, however, later declare the unavailability of safer sexual practices which reduce transmission of infectious disease. Only gay men's sexual abstinence, they say, can stop this scourge.

This is indicative of the smeared queer—situated on the border of sex and disease. Since Sohn and Robilotti characterize male homosexuality to be an illness in their coining of gay bowel syndrome, abstinence can possibly prevent it. In order to prevent gay bowel syndrome, one could prevent the continuation of same-sex sexual activity. Forget about condoms and other barrier devices, monogamy, or nonpenetrative sexual practices. Such statements that "the only safer sex is no sex at all" would take on considerable significance with the later onslaught of HIV infections.

In addition, gay bowel syndrome is at times regarded as invisible or not immediately apparent. A lack of symptoms was noted by several researchers as especially dangerous due to epidemiological concerns of bringing the illness under control once identified. "The existence of such a carrier state implies that once the agent is introduced into a community, a reservoir of infection will continue to exist even if all symptomatic patients are quickly identified and treated."[41] In this way, all gay men become potential carriers of gay bowel syndrome pathogens. Homosexuality becomes effectively homogenized as the contradictory symptom of a nonsymptomatic pathology, and no gay man, regardless of how healthy he might feel or appear, is able to escape scientific and popular suspicion. The homosexual male becomes a public health outlaw, necessitating a special surveillance, for only careful monitoring enabled by medical technology can distinguish between the suspect and the criminal.

IN THE BOWELS OF THE OTHER

In 1983, a writer for *The New York Times* mapped a perceived invasion of foreign contagion in an article entitled "AIDS: A New Disease's Deadly Odyssey," identifying an urban gay neighborhood as the geography of infestation. "Indeed, bizarre infections are so common in the homosexual community that one [unnamed] scientist, presenting a report on these occurrences in 1968, called his talk, 'Manhattan: The Tropical Isle.' "[42] In chronicling the cross of contagion gay men have supposedly learned to bear, Dennis L. Breo wrote in a 1987 *Chicago Tribune* article, "They also learned to endure the rare intestinal parasites of 'the gay bowel syndrome,' a variety of discomforting diseases, like salmonella, that are normally confined to tropical islands."[43]

Gay bowel syndrome becomes a highly effective tool for the "Othering" of gay men in many respects, apart from a basic distinction between gay men's bowels and heterosexual men's bowels in a diseased/healthy dichotomy. The syndrome also constructs gay men as physiological foreigners and aliens—tropical, animalistic, primitive, and unsanitary. Gay bowel syndrome tells us not only what medicine believes (and creates) gay men to be in the scientific and popular minds, but how Western science imagines itself (and the general population) in relation to the third world, the precivilized, the nonhuman, and the unhygienic.

As early as the 1960s, many tropical parasites not commonly found in people living in North America and considered to be endemic in tropical regions were realized to be sexually transmittable. Diagnoses of several of these tropical parasites in gay men who had not traveled abroad conveniently served as consequential evidence of perversity, combining the decadence of the primitive with the evils of the exotic and ancient sexual practices of analingus and anal intercourse. These parasites also enable a vision of the gay bowel as a frighteningly diversified garden, plush and rich in its mysteriously dangerous flora and fauna, an overpluralized ecology of imported microbiological immigrants. The gay bowel becomes a multinational melting pot representing transgressed boundaries, a vessel for foreign invaders who endanger public wellness. The tropical bowel defines gay men to be cesspools of morbidity while staking a public claim of necessary intervention for the sake of the common good. The tropical alien therefore must be contained, watched, regulated, and vilified.

Apart from the hegemonic Othering of gay men as tropically infested, nationalism plays a strong role among gay medical authorities in terms of origin stories and attribution of the spread of these diseases. In the pages of *The Advocate*, Randy Shilts paraphrases Dan Williams' description of the chain of infection from other countries to gay men in the United States:

Williams thinks the diseases are first appearing in the major port cities because of the large tropical populations common to those areas. These populations bring the disease into the country and then spread them into the gay communities. From the time it hits the gay communities of these gay meccas, it's only a matter of time before it plays to the inland gay crowds, many gay health authorities warn.[44]

The unnamed tropical populations are said to have spread these diseases into gay communities. Exactly how did this spread occur—and why only into gay communities? If transmission was through sexual activity, then why are these "tropical populations" considered to be apart from gay communities. The language clearly suggests disease was spread into gay male populations, not among or within. The implication is that gay community really means the white, Western, United States, economically advantaged gay community. This perceived chain of infection results in an imbrication of Otherness—an overlapping series of infectious Others each in contact with the next, yet paradoxically distinct in separation. This creates a cartography of xenophobic sexual access through simultaneous recognitions and denials of sleeping with the Other.

Building upon this Otherness of the tropics and foreign nationality, conceptualizations of third world poverty and unsanitary conditions have also been used by popular media to vilify the diseased gay bowel. A 1987 *Chicago Tribune* article quips, "As a group, the promiscuous gays have more kinds of pathogenic, or potentially pathogenic, bacteria in their intestines than a Bangladeshi peasant" and quotes Joseph Sonnabend, a pathologist with the Uniformed University of the Health Sciences, as saying, "This exposure to many different enteric organisms [in reference to 1970s Greenwich Village promiscuity] can create in homosexual communities a situation similar to that found in nations where primitive sanitary facilities result in endemic infections."[45] Images of unsanitary conditions, malnutrition, and primitiveness all enter this enteric picture through cross-global and cross-species connections drawn by popular media. Pearl Ma, microbiology chief at St. Vincent's Hospital in New York City, was quoted in a 1982 United Press International newswire story as stating that "Gay bowel syndrome is extremely rare in the United States because it is caused by a tropical parasite found in countries with poor sanitation."[46]

The article continues by recounting Ma's need to adapt a common veterinarian's test for examination of feces to detect parasites and bacteria in order to find the syndrome in the St. Vincent's patients. Gay bowel syndrome in this article is defined to be "where intestinal infections caused by bacteria and parasites associated with animals are found in humans."[47] Not only are gay men considered unsanitary, but they are so primitive (perhaps due to their "evolutionary slumming") that they share microorganisms with nonhumans. Zoonoses, which include not only parasites but ebola virus and simian herpes, are defined as diseases crossing from nature to man and vice versa, usually as the result of a laboratory accident or a primitive practice that is thought to violate the boundaries of the natural.[48]

AIDS AND GAY BOWEL SYNDROME: CAUSATION, CORRELATION, AND CONFLATION

In the early 1980s, the emergence of acquired immune system disorders was often described by the Centers for Disease Control and other medical authorities as occurring in "previously healthy" gay men. In *Inventing AIDS*, Cindy Patton argues that the medical view of pre-AIDS gay men as healthy, despite commonly having a variety of sexually transmitted diseases,

> attested to the acceptance and positive valuation of gay men and their sexuality in the urban settings where these early [AIDS] cases were under study. Had these cases appeared fifty years ago, and had the homosexuality of the patients been recognized [in that hypothetical time period], doctors would probably have viewed homosexuals *per se* as constitutionally weaker and explained their immune system breakdown on this fact alone.[49]

In consideration of the metaphors attached to gay bowel syndrome, and considering that the syndrome emerged from medical practices in the hearts of urban gay ghettos, we see that one need not reimagine a time of five decades past, but simply look to the late 1970s to see Patton's and several other cultural theorists' oversight. Gay men were in fact considered to be anything but "previously healthy." For it is precisely in gay bowel syndrome discourse that we discover these medical scientists' view of gay constitutional weakness in the homosexual body; and gay men's acquired immune system breakdowns were often correlated with, attributed to, and conflated with gay bowel syndrome. This important link has been widely neglected in contemporary theoretical works seeking to gain deeper understandings of AIDS metaphors, signifiers, origin stories, and discursive practices.

In *And the Band Played On*, Randy Shilts documented that in June 1981, the Kaposi's Sarcoma and Opportunistic Infections (KSOI) Task Force (which Shilts called a "medical detective agency") in Atlanta pulled together an interdisciplinary team of medical researchers which included parasitologists due to the suspicion that gay bowel syndrome might be intrinsically linked to the appearance of new immune system disorders found in gay men.[50] From the earliest investigations of what would later be named AIDS, gay bowel syndrome was an important consideration in terms of causation and correlation. On December 21, 1981, *Time* magazine reported a puzzling new syndrome of opportunistic diseases in gay men, speculating an immunologic overload theory in part due to intestinal disruptions caused by gay bowel syndrome. San Francisco physician Robert Bolan is quoted in the article as speculating, "This constant, chronic stimulation to their [homosexual men's] immune system may eventually cause the system to collapse."[51]

Many historians and other theorists mark the coining of the term GRID (gay-related immune deficiency) as the pivotal event that popularized the notion of gay-specific disease (in both name and application) not purely psychological in nature. As we have seen, however, not only does gay bowel syndrome predate GRID, but it sets the stage for GRID's debut and paves the way for the construction of AIDS as the second gay disease. The earliest textual evidence of the use of GRID comes from a paper presented at a conference of the American Federation for Clinical Research in Washington, DC, in May 1982. The abstract of the paper, "Gay-Related Immunodeficiency (GRID) Syndrome: Clinical and Autopsy Observations," by Michael Gottlieb and his four associates, offers findings from the examination of ten individuals with severe T-cell dysfunction and multiple opportunistic infections. Despite the gay-specific title of the paper, these researchers admit that of the ten patients, "Eight were homosexual; two were exclusively heterosexual."[52] As with gay bowel syndrome, GRID was built upon a generalization which later stigmatized an entire population.

Names other than GRID, AIDS, and ACIDS (acquired immuno-deficiency syndrome) included CAID—Community Acquired Immunodeficiency,[53] Gay Cancer,[54] Homosexual Syndrome,[55] Gay Lymph-Node Syndrome,[56] and Homosexual Compromise Syndrome.[57] The naming of these diseases as being community acquired and gay-specific indicates a social relation between a particular culture and the biological domain of nature, two entities popularly imagined to be separate and distinct from each other. Both GRID and gay bowel syndrome serve as useful conceptual mechanisms in the ways in which they create a tense traffic between essentialist and constructionist ideas of identity and disease, nature and culture, and language and the body. *The* gay community becomes essentialized in this respect as an ethnic identity through a grounding in epidemiology. Thus the coining and formulation of gay diseases solidifies and enhances the essentialization of individuals sharing a same-sex sexual preference. Similarly, the conceptualization of gay ethnicity, identity, and community lends itself to essentialist conceptions of diseases, in this case gay plagues. As Steven Epstein states, "The deaths of middle-class, white, gay men attracted more medical attention, and because of that, and because gays were seen as a sort of ethnic group, AIDS first became known as a 'gay disease.'"[58]

Media representations furthering the conflation between GRID and gay bowel syndrome became increasingly common in the early 1980s. In 1982, a United Press International article reported on the annual meeting of the Tennessee Medical Association which included a presentation on Kaposi's sarcoma by William Schaffner of Vanderbilt University School of Medicine. Schaffner definitively tied Kaposi's sarcoma, a rare cancer previously found in elderly men of Mediterranean descent but now emerging in younger gay men, to gay bowel syndrome. The article reports with certainty, "The cancerous tumor is linked to a collection of infections called gay bowel syndrome, contracted mostly by homosexual men."[59] In an August

1983 *New York Native* article speculating on the possible causes of AIDS, Dr. Richard Pearce stated, "Chronic or multiple parasitic infections alone could account for the immunosuppression associated with AIDS."[60] In a follow-up feature later that year, Pearce proposed, "I believe that of all these assaults to the immune system [exposure to sperm, ultraviolet irradiation, drug use, lack of sleep, and STDs], parasitic [intestinal] infections are the major, *if not sole*, risk factor for acquired immune deficiency syndrome."[61] Although the term gay bowel syndrome is never invoked here, the chronic and multiple nature of these intestinal infections certainly fits within the syndrome's general definition. As recently as June 1993 in an *American Spectator* feature titled "Rethinking HIV," writer Tom Bethell argued the cause of AIDS is not HIV, but rather a "gay lifestyle," which includes, among other things, fisting, rectal injuries, rimming, and of course gay bowel syndrome.[62]

Gay bowel syndrome slowly moved from the category of possible AIDS cause or cofactor to that of an item subsumed under the AIDS laundry list of opportunistic diseases. One 1988 study attempted to demonstrate that HIV-infected gay men are more likely than HIV-negative gay men to have gay bowel syndrome as an opportunistic infection.[63] Gay bowel syndrome has in this way become a possible syndrome within a syndrome, a microcosm of a larger smeared, run together picture. But since HIV-positive people are, as a group, more prone to having *any* opportunistic infection than HIV-negative people, the conclusion would seem obvious. Within this syndromic framework, homosexuality is an underlying process contributing not only to the constitution of disease, but to HIV infection as well.

Gay bowel syndrome set the stage for future AIDS politics in many other ways. The tropical nature of gay contagion found in gay bowel syndrome discourse was also a precursor for additional forms of AIDS-Othering. Not only did this help to lay the groundwork for the Haiti/AIDS connection six years later, but it made excellent background music to Randy Shilts's soap operatic narrative of French-Canadian airline attendant Gaetan (Patient Zero) Dugas's demonic sexual tourism. [64] Shilts's journalism has become such a strong thread connecting gay bowel syndrome and AIDS, in fact, that a 1994 two-page "in memoriam" article on Shilts in the

Journal of Sex Research credited and highlighted Shilts's deliverance of gay bowel syndrome medical news to the public at large. The author of the tribute reflects,

> In retrospect, this short story about an increasing number of highly unusual cases of sexually transmitted disease [gay bowel syndrome] can be read as a prolegomenon to a tragic tale of disease and despair that would shortly follow.[65]

Gay bowel syndrome is historicized here as a prediction for the plague to come, a warning sign interpreted and brought forth by Shilts as the prophet.[66] If only we had paid more attention, we lament. If only we had listened to the Truth of Medicine and learned our lesson from gay bowel syndrome. A particular righteousness is in this way endowed to gay bowel syndrome—we must fear it, we must believe in it, we must acknowledge the power of devastation it possesses, for we have seen what happens when we fail to do so.

In terms of heeding the messages of HIV-prevention campaigns, gay men were often criticized for their resistance to medical authoritative attempts to close bath houses and regulate same-sex sexual practices in the early 1980s. In understanding the political role played by gay bowel syndrome just prior to the invention of GRID, one might gain particular insight into one case where such mistrust originated, and the validity of resistant action toward those who had already stated that the only safer gay male sex is complete abstinence. For example, as the Sohn and Robilotti article suggested, no chemical or mechanical prophylaxes were believed to work in the prevention of an existing gay-specific disease, why should it work for this new one?

THE HOMOSEXUAL MENACE: GAY BOWEL SYNDROME AS GROUNDS FOR ANTIGAY DISCRIMINATION

The use of gay bowel syndrome as a justification for antigay discrimination and inequality has consistently entered civil rights debates surrounding gay men and lesbian women in the last twenty years. Such arenas of contestation that gay bowel syndrome has entered include: the proposed 1994 Federal Employment Non-

Discrimination Act which would have prohibited employment discrimination on the basis of sexual orientation,[67] the gays in the military debate, the Cracker Barrel restaurant chain's decision to adopt a policy banning employment of gay and lesbian individuals, California state legislation targeting gay men for mandatory reporting and contact tracing of infectious diseases, the inclusion of a gay teenage character in the nationally syndicated comic strip *For Better or Worse,* the 1994 Colorado Amendment 2 proceedings, and arguments over the suitability of gay and lesbian couples as adoptive parents.

Andrew Plaut, a gastrointestinal specialist at Tufts University New England Medical Center in Boston, in a 1982 UPI story, is paraphrased as saying that "bisexual men who come into the cities for several sexual contacts a night and return to their wives may be spreading the disease among heterosexuals" and that gay bowel syndrome "is the latest link in what the doctors fear is a contagion that could reach heterosexuals."[68] The implicit warning in this passage is the forecast that gay bowel syndrome might spread into the general population. Jan Zita Grover illuminates how the general population is set up in relation to high risk groups and AIDS:

> According to the term's users—the media, public health officials, politicians—"the general population" is virtuously going about its business, which is not pleasure-seeking (as drugs and gay life are uniformly imagined to be), so AIDS hits its members as an assault from diseased hedonists upon hard-working innocents.[69]

Plaut's statement is also unique in that it complicates a clear distinction between the innocent general population and the guilty high-risk group. This appears to be the only instance of directly mentioning bisexuality to be of import in the transmission of gay bowel syndrome conditions. Plaut, unlike other writers, tells his readers exactly how gay bowel syndrome might cross over from the perverts to the morally clean, resulting in a process of innocent infection. Anyone can be susceptible to the medical consequences of homosexuality, instilling fear and panic as a motivator for discriminatory practices, homophobic violence, and oppression.

The early conflations between gay bowel syndrome and AIDS were sometimes noted by those who used both terms in substantiating denial of civil rights to gay, lesbian, and bisexual people. In a 1983 *Time* letter to the editor, Pat Buchanan expresses his dissatisfaction in being misquoted in regard to gay diseases:

> In your article, you left the impression that I had recommended that active homosexuals be "barred" from the foodhandling business because of AIDS. Not so. The danger from homosexual food handlers is not AIDS, but the spread of enteric diseases (the so-called gay bowel syndrome), several of which are epidemic among gays and are spread by contaminated food.[70]

Buchanan himself is quick to make this careful distinction between the gay diseases he speaks of, enumerating the possibilities of several gay diseases that the public should remain vigilant and wary of, although he ultimately conflates them.

Other than bisexuality, food handling is the major threat of gay bowel syndrome cross contagion. Ed McAteer, president of the Religious Roundtable on *Larry King Live* (December 2, 1991), "That's one of the reasons that I'm for the Cracker Barrel people, because it's reliably reported that the majority of gay men have what is called gay bowel disease and it's a contagious disease and people handling foods—That can be transmitted." Larry King then asked a follow-up question for clarification, "Under that concept, then, no homosexual should be employed around the public?" McAteer replies, "Absolutely—not food handling, especially." The relationship between the vulnerably healthy heterosexual and the threat of diseased others is one of anxiety-ridden imagination where the exotic foreigner spreads diseases into gay men who, stereotypically employed as waiters and food handlers, either contaminate the food of the unsuspecting heterosexual restaurant patron or donate blood and taint the life source of our nation's blood supply.

In a 1994 *Washington Times* article, Karen Jo Gounaud wrote, "Another consequence of male-male sex is a rise in 'gay bowel syndrome,' a condition contributing to serious health and hygiene problems."[71] This statement is culled from a larger news piece supporting a local library's decision to purchase antigay books, and she dubs her argument "the Truth of Natural Consequences." By 1994 it was no longer publicly acceptable to say AIDS is a gay disease, but one can still refer to another gay disease as evidence of homosexual danger—gay bowel syndrome. Gounaud sets up male-male sex to be unnatural, then attempts to logically conclude the punitive consequences for violating nature.

In response to an article addressing the need for legal recognition of same-sex couples, a letter appeared in the February 1995 issue of the *National Law Journal* by a distressed and concerned man stating that,

> According to an article in *American Family Medicine*, an entire group of intestinal diseases are so common among the homosexual population that they are referred to collectively as "gay bowel syndrome." . . . Your newspaper would not consider encouraging lawyers or legal staff to live an alcoholic lifestyle, a narcotic lifestyle or a criminal lifestyle. There is no reason to support the homosexual lifestyle, which is just as destructive to its participants.[72]

The authority of science is invoked as conclusive evidence and objective truth, complete with a citation for its textual source. The writer moves the issue of sexual politics from a legal and moral plane to that of an essentialist investigation, artificially segregating nature from culture in denial of the traffic between the two.

In 1991, Congressman William Dannemeyer wrote a column for the *Chicago Tribune* on the hotly contested issue of gays in the military:

> But if you need a rational basis to discriminate, there is one. Male homosexuals are generally one of the unhealthiest groups of people on record. Long before AIDS, homosexuals routinely suffered from a multitude of venereal diseases with names like gay bowel syndrome. . .[73]

These comments by Dannemeyer came on the heels of his earlier book *Shadow in the Land: Homosexuality in America*, in which he discusses gay bowel syndrome. "GBS is a complex of symptoms (fever, diarrhea, etc.) that first occurred in a number of California homosexuals and later spread throughout the country, eventually infecting heterosexuals as well."[74] Congressman Dannemeyer offers a quite different origin story of gay bowel syndrome with a traffic pattern stemming from the West coast and radiating outward to encompass even heterosexuals. This story serves to trace the medical and moral menace of gay bowel syndrome to California and, presumably, San Francisco in particular. His "shadow in the land" is cast from the homosexual community of decadent California that spreads its all-consuming pallor eastward across the country.

These rationalizations are most creatively exemplified by the title of a 1990 pamphlet, authored by Paul Cameron and published by the right-wing neoconservative Family Research Institute, *Medical Consequences of What Homosexuals Do.* Cameron ominously warns unsuspecting straights and queers alike of the dangers of same-sex sexual behaviors in his speeches, presentations, and legislative testimony around the country. Cameron cooks up biohazards of anal sex as a recipe for disaster. With the rectum as its "mixing bowl," Cameron offers for our consumption of disdain the multi-ingredient, polymicrobial gay bowel syndrome as a prime example of homosexual doom.[75]

When editor in chief Ian Haysom defended the 1993 decision to continue printing the comic strip *For Better or Worse* in the *Vancouver Sun* amid the controversy of the strip's positive depiction of a gay teenager, reader Trevor Lautens responded fiercely in an editorial printed by the newspaper. Haysom had advised parents, "Instead of rushing to hide the comic section . . . I'd suggest you answer your kids' questions as honestly and openly as you can." Lauten countered, "Those parents Haysom counsels better be able to tell their children not only about AIDS but also about the sometimes deadly hepatitis B. About gay bowel syndrome. About all the other diseases of Latinate terms that arise from a simple fact: the human anus is not a safe vessel for the human penis."[76] The theme of "unnatural anus as poor substitute for natural vagina" appears once again here, as well as the implication that anal penetration by the human penis is assaultive, violent, and necessarily causes disease.

In June 1995, Samuel P. Woodward, president of Citizens Alliance of Washington, authored an editorial printed in *The Columbian* newspaper. He discussed in great detail the substantiated denial of rights to gay and lesbian people wishing to adopt children or provide foster care:

> Homosexuals' lifestyle makes them the most efficient trans-
> mitter of all sexually transmitted diseases. . . . They *enjoy* high
> rates of infection from cytomegalovirus, amoebic bowel dis-
> ease and a cluster of infections collectively referred to as "gay
> bowel syndrome."[77] (Italics mine)

The choice of the word "enjoy" in reference to suffering from disease is a curious one, although not surprising since it neatly ties back into the equation of disease and hedonistic homo pleasures. That lesbian women are also presumably included in the homosex-ual lifestyle is also somewhat of an inaccuracy, for no medical texts using gay bowel syndrome apply the diagnosis to women who have sex with women. There is also an underlying assumption that one must be completely free of disease in order to be a competent parent, so this naturally excludes anyone performing perverse sex-ual acts.

The above passages are but a sampling of the deployment of gay bowel syndrome in efforts to deny queer people equality in employ-ment, parenting, service in the military, positive media representa-tion, and more. The breadth of political issues into which gay bowel syndrome enters indicates the multivariant utility of such a term—concrete enough to refer, but vague enough to be applicable to virtually any argument regarding sexual preference. The antigay radical right accelerates its political movements by translating gay bowel syndrome medical journal articles to the public, without contextualizing the creation of the term in the late 1970s or discuss-ing its position within medical discourse. Unfortunately, gay men have not, at this time, articulated a forceful or effective response to this maneuver, complicated as it may be.

CONCLUSIONS

One question remains: Why was the term GRID so vehemently challenged and soon after eradicated, while the term gay bowel syndrome continues to be used so extensively? Gay bowel syndrome has appeared in literature as recently as 1999, including a 1993 STD educational brochure.[78] Challenges to the deployment of gay bowel syndrome, as a term or a practical concept, are almost nonexistent. It is important to note here that in most gay periodicals, such as *The Advocate*, *New York Native*, and *Gay Community News*, the term gay bowel syndrome is never used in the text of the articles when referring to these sexually transmitted diseases affecting the anus and rectum, although gay bowel syndrome medical journal articles are endnoted or cited at the end. This careful avoidance indicates gay journalists' wariness of the term, but within this suspicious silence they fail to state why the term is less than preferable and likewise do not call for the abandonment of its use. Even in a 1984 *New York Native* article titled "The New Medical Journal Homophobia," which explores both overt as well as more subtle homophobia in scientific literature used by physicians to perpetuate their own cultural bigotry, author James D'Eramo fails to even once mention gay bowel syndrome.

Some possible reasons for this silence might be that gay bowel syndrome was not depicted to be as fatal or mysterious in etiology as GRID; therefore the stakes might not have been as high in the minds of progay activists, rightfully concentrating on other issues of survival. A sense of urgency might have prioritized attention to GRID in a time of increasing gay male morbidity. Additionally, in the case of GRID, the Centers for Disease Control took leadership and officially named the syndrome AIDS, and even offered a fairly extensive, formal definition of what the government considered to be AIDS.

Another reason might be the Randy Shilts-esque parable of the disregarded herald mentioned earlier. To some extent this cast a grim shadow over attempts to eliminate the term, for if gay bowel syndrome was the unheeded harbinger of plague, a cultural wariness wells up within those who would exorcise this particular demon. Gay bowel syndrome is in some ways granted this respect for its fable of malignant neglect.

Of the multitude of arenas in which gay bowel syndrome appears, only two strong and direct challenges materialize. During a 1983 symposium on AIDS held at New York University Medical Center, Roger Enlow and Ron Grossman emphasized medical ethics in the treatment of gay patients, pointing out that, "just as Legionnaires' disease and 'the gay bowel syndrome' were inappropriately named, we must not consider AIDS a 'gay disease.'" Grossman followed up with the statement, "Let us not cloak ourselves behind icy technology," encouraging a mindfulness of the human dimensions of disease and tragedy and challenging medical bigotry masked in technologies of purported scientific truth.[79]

In a rare and bold challenge to the use of the term gay bowel syndrome in a 1993 *American Family Physician* article, four physicians in a residency program in social medicine at Montefiore Medical Center in the Bronx—Rick O'Keefe, Peter Marcus, Janet Townshend, and Marji Gold—authored a letter to the editor. They disputed, "the infections listed . . . in the article are not exclusive to homosexual males but are found in people with human immunodeficiency virus (HIV) infection or in those who practice unprotected anal sex."[80] They continued by stating that gay men who are not HIV positive and do not practice unprotected anal sex may be subjected to unnecessary diagnostic tests simply because of their sexual orientation. They cited the additional danger of misdiagnosis in an example of a twenty-five-year-old gay man whose symptoms of colon cancer were misdiagnosed as gay bowel syndrome, despite his strong family history of early colon cancer.

Their letter is met with an icy reply, in which the authors of the original article, Hastings and Weber, justify their use of the term by countering,

> The term not only identifies a *high-risk group* likely to manifest the syndrome, it also suggests a specific group of pathogenic organisms for which to look. Although the term gay bowel syndrome may lack the *"political sensitivity"* of the terms suggested by Dr. O'Keefe and colleagues, the term is nevertheless more descriptive and precise than the alternatives.[81] (Italics mine)

Addressing the case of misdiagnosed colon cancer, they reply, "The case of the homosexual patient with colon cancer misdiagnosed as gay bowel disease seems to be one of inappropriate medical evaluation rather than inappropriate nomenclature."[82] This statement implies the body exists as a conceptual entity wholly apart from the names which represent its conditions. Hastings and Weber refuse to recognize that the name of an illness can blind or mislead medical practitioners to the causes and consequences of the symptoms they are dealing with. Just because a misdiagnosis occurred does not mean the diagnostic classification system failed the physician, they argue, but only that the physician failed the system.

Use of the phrase high-risk group rather than an emphasis on high-risk behavior as late as 1993 should be evidence enough of these researchers' need to cling to scapegoating rhetoric and blame-the-victim mentality. Jan Zita Grover discusses at length the concept of risk group and the functions it serves:

> In the media and in political debate, the epidemiological category of risk group has been used to stereotype and stigmatize people already seen as outside the moral and economic parameters of the "general population." . . . [This] makes clear the social and political, as opposed to epidemiological, functions of the risk group concept: to isolate and condemn people rather than to contact and protect them.[83]

The comment that gay bowel syndrome might lack political sensitivity but is more precise than other terminology attempts to draw clear and rigid boundaries between the realms of politics and science, as if the two are separate entities which do not impact each other. Hastings and Weber chastise their challengers for dissolving this boundary and concerning themselves with the subjectivity and humanity (i.e., sensitivity) of the political ramifications beyond the sphere of the hospital or clinic.

The history and progression of gay bowel syndrome as a scientific fact is certainly disturbing and complicated. It set the stage for GRID and AIDS from 1976 to 1980, even though no one knew it would do so at the time. One is left with a series of "what ifs," pondering the continuing development of gay diseases had HIV never entered the scene. Perhaps gay bowel syndrome would have faded into medical journal obscurity if it had not been conveniently revived in attempts to explain gay male immune deficiencies and substantiate oppression in a time of increasing fear and hatred directed toward gay men as a form of blame for the AIDS pandemic.

I view this thesis as a first step in the work necessary to facilitate the debunking of gay bowel syndrome as an acceptable epidemiological term and appropriate diagnostic practice. This will be no simple feat of linguistic stylechange, however. Although I have chosen to focus primarily on the United States here, the term gay bowel syndrome has been exported for use worldwide, already having appeared in medical journals in Australia,[84] Sweden,[85] Germany,[86] England,[87] Belgium,[88] and Puerto Rico.[89] The ramifications of this dissemination should not be underestimated as merely the semantic adoption of technical jargon. The possibility that gay bowel syndrome could be used in devastating ways to oppress gay men around the world is quite frightening. Differing cultural concepts of gay, health, disease, and medicine will determine exactly how gay bowel syndrome will unfold in these countries.

We must rename gay bowel syndrome if we truly believe it to be a constellation of conditions requiring a formal referent or we must cease use of the term and rely upon differential diagnoses. It is possible to conceptualize these illnesses and conditions without lumping them together and branding the package with a gay name. Physicians can still be trained to treat gay male patients effectively and reasonably consider diseases found to be of high incidence among gay male populations. With more description and clarity, differential diagnoses such as inflammatory bowel disease or proctitis can serve as advantageous signifiers for bodily conditions requiring treatment and professional care. This is a practical, concrete instance of an attempt to disentangle homosexuality and disease.

I do not support eradication of the notion and use of gay disease altogether, however. Activists and writers such as Simon Watney, Edward King, Michael Callen, Eric Rofes, and others have repeatedly articulated the need for a gay AIDS.[90] The de-gaying of AIDS, beginning around 1985, and the recent attempts to re-gay AIDS have been met with great ambivalence and controversy, however. The crux of this positioning is a focus on the difference between saying "AIDS is not a gay disease" and "AIDS is not *just* a gay disease." The well-intentioned, knee-jerk reaction to mid-1980s homophobic equations of HIV infection and homosexuality, coupled with an avid concern over rising rates of HIV infection in nongay populations, has resulted in the marginalization and neglect of gay men in efforts of

AIDS education, prevention, care provision, visibility, and funding. Much of the 1985 de-gaying of AIDS represented an attempt to find ways to talk about HIV infection outside, as well as inside, gay male communities, to refashion the meaning of language for people living with HIV regardless of the way they became infected.[91]

Despite the value in the notion of some forms of gay disease, gay bowel syndrome yields few, if any, productive or insightful benefits for gay men. An analysis of the construction of scientific knowledge (in this case, gay bowel syndrome) reveals anxieties based on homophobic cultural values, numerous self-contradictions, and the popularization of gay bowel syndrome and other gay diseases after the onset of AIDS. Gay bowel syndrome is a self-contradictory construction supporting an essentialized category of difference that simply cannot be applied to all anorectal diseases as a syndrome, all gay men as a typology, nor to all anal practices as unhealthy. These hazy definitions of gay bowel syndrome provide an ideal entrypoint for disruption and a call for its abandonment. Use of the term gay bowel syndrome must be nullified before it further lends itself to the formation of social policies and governing practices that seek to force gay male bodies into positions of social, cultural, medical, and political subordination.

SECTION II:
SMEARING TO SPREAD
A WET SUBSTANCE

The Plumber's Applause

I was working
the clinic
when you'd caught
more than my eye.
So handsome
in the waiting room,
I said, "Fix that
drip,
and we'll talk."
You and your plumbing
left the building
with penicillin
and my number.
But *someone* can't
follow instructions
and now your mild
clap
has become
my standing ovation.

Chapter 2

Gay Men and the Female Condom:
Is Rectal Reality Getting a Bum Wrap?

In a time when sexual activity relies heavily upon technologies that make physical contact safer from disease transmission, the availability and use of HIV-antibody tests, latex and polyurethane barriers, and vaginal and anal microbicides have acquired increasingly significant roles since the early 1980s. The commodification and diversification of these devices have also dramatically increased as they have become necessary goods for many sexually active people who seek to reduce their risk of HIV infection. The process of diversification in this area has given rise to gender-specific safer sex products, developed for two general reasons: (1) Manufacturers are able to target consumer populations that constitute a market niche, and (2) public health officials have called for scientifically engineered technologies that are tailored to female bodies in an effort to curb the rate of new HIV infections. The emergence of these gendered products has not been without controversy, however. While they continue to serve the basic function of a physical barrier to pathogens, the widespread implications of these technologies' impact on human relations have only begun to be realized.

Perhaps the most notorious of these devices is the Reality Female Condom. From the time of its introduction to the United States, Reality has been a consistent source of contention related to gender and sexuality. The device calls into question relations of power in ways that threaten to shift the norms and enablement of technologized sexual practices. Gay men's recent appropriation of this "female" condom for same-sex anal intercourse, represents one of the most intense and dramatic of these shifts. It reveals the dangers of crossing gendered lines that have traditionally been constructed and enforced through systems of government regulation, consumer capitalism, and scientific invention, among others.

At the time of this writing, we are more than seventeen years into the AIDS epidemic, and not a single condom has been officially approved by the United States government for anal sex. In a time when gay men struggle to maintain their safer sex practices, some have become desperate for alternative devices that preserve or enhance the pleasures of penetrative sexual activity. Despite a lack of government approval, some gay men have chosen Reality Female Condom as that alternative. Although versions of the male condom have existed for hundreds of years, Reality is the first sexual barrier device to radically depart from the traditional design of a sheath worn on the penis. Because it is an artifice that is applied internally rather than externally to the body, it has attracted attention as something of a sexual oddity. Reality's savvy packaging boasts the ability to prevent unwanted pregnancy and sexually transmitted infection, while simultaneously claiming to endow its user with greater gendered equality by balancing the scales of control between insertive and receptive partners of heterosexual intercourse.

Reality is no longer a device configured solely for female receptive sex partners, however. On the contrary, Reality's ease of appropriation actually takes on a form of agency as it demands configuration of both the male and female users who are most desperate for the alternatives and possibilities it affords them. In many ways, the prescribed relationship between user and technological device is akin to that between gender and sexual behavior. Both sets of relations come with a package of instructions, rewards for compliance, and punishments for deviation. But both can be disrupted and disruptive. Devices and sexual acts can be subverted and perverted; users and genders can be fluid and malleable. These two analogous interplays between device and user, and between gender and sexuality, can be comparatively traced and analyzed through the unique challenges that Reality poses to policy makers, AIDS prevention specialists, private corporations, religious organizations, medical professionals, and sexually active individuals.

In her book, *Bodies That Matter*, philosopher Judith Butler states that, "In psychoanalytic terms, the relation between gender and sexuality is in part negotiated through the question of identification and desire. And here it becomes clear why refusing to draw lines of causal implication between these two domains is as important as keeping open an investigation of their complex interimplication."[1] Butler continues by describing an imaginary logic of heterosexuality that attempts to masquerade as the norm of reality, "For, if to identify as a woman is not necessarily to desire a man, and if to desire a woman does not necessarily signal the constituting presence of a masculine identification, whatever that is, then the heterosexual matrix proves to be an imaginary logic that insistently issues forth its own unmanageability."[2] Herein lies the irony of the female condom's unmanageable controversies, for they include an imaginary heterosexual reality and a Reality that, by its own appropriated use, exposes and signifies the artificiality of this imagination.

The debates that continue to rage around Reality, in conjunction with the suspicious silences that dictate its market survival, serve as predictions for the inevitable complications in future development and application of gender-specific HIV-prevention technologies. They also lend a greater understanding of the relationship between technologies and human lives. The collision of material bodies, gendered sex acts, and sexually enabling devices provoke heightened anxieties surrounding the appropriation of technology for unapproved and unintended use while clearly marking the boundaries of gender even as they are sexually transgressed.

HISTORICAL REALITY

Invented by a Danish physician in 1984, Reality has been widely available in European countries since 1992. In the fall of 1987, Wisconsin Pharmacal Company (WPC) licensed the marketing rights from Chartex International for sale of the female condom in the United States and Canada. In the United States, the device received approval from the Food and Drug Administration (FDA) and was accessible for over-the-counter purchase by late 1994, packaged as the "Reality female condom" by the Female Health Company, a division of WPC. The female condom is a polyurethane sheath with a plastic ring on each end. The sheath itself is six and one-half inches long and three inches wide. The inner ring is loose inside the sheath, with a diameter of two inches. The outer ring forms the rim of the sheath's opening with a diameter of two and three quarter inches. When inserted into the vagina, the inner ring is anchored against the pubic bone while the outer ring remains outside the body and keeps the entire device from being inserted and lost.

Clinical trials of Reality have involved more than 1,700 heterosexual couples using 30,000 devices in ten countries. Some of these tests involved distribution of Reality to women through family planning clinics in Latin America.

While under FDA scrutiny, a study conducted in the United States with 200 hundred women found Reality to have a 26 percent failure rate of pregnancy prevention. James Trussel, a medical consultant for Reality from Princeton University, explained to the Associated Press, however, that the 26 percent failure rate included sexual acts in which couples did not use Reality at all. He also stated that, "With perfect use—with each act of intercourse—the female condom has a failure rate of only 5 percent, compared to 3 percent for the male condom."[3] The FDA gave its lukewarm approval of Reality after fast-tracking the study of 200 women for six months, as compared to the usual full year of study, citing the urgency of additional options needed for HIV protection.

In 1991, prior to FDA approval, the Female Health Company commissioned the Howard Brown Memorial Clinic in Chicago to conduct clinical research of the device's appropriateness for male-to-male anal sex. The two principal investigators were Robert G. Jobst, MD, and Judith S. Johns, RN, MSN. They prepared an unpublished report of their findings titled, "Investigation of an Inserted Anal Condom (Aegis) for the Receptive Partner Involved in Anal Sex." The tentative brand name of the device at that time was "Aegis," and was sometimes referred to by WPC as a condom and at other times a barrier pouch. According to Jobst and Johns, the stated objectives of the clinic's study were threefold: to ascertain whether the Aegis concept was acceptable to gay males engaging in anal sex, to determine the condom's protective capability, and to gauge the condom's comfort and compatibility.[4]

The acceptability of Reality was defined from two perspectives: how well it performed during anal intercourse in terms of breakage and dislodgment, and the overall acceptance as an alternative to the traditional male latex condom from both the insertive and receptive user's viewpoint.

Gay male couples were recruited in the Chicago area through advertisements in gay publications and brochures in gay-oriented businesses. In order to be eligible for the study, the couples were required to possess the following characteristics: between sixteen and fifty years of age, monogamous, sexually active and participating in anal sex, free of any sexually transmitted infections, no known allergy to latex or polyurethane, free of penile and anal abrasions, and must have passed a general physical examination. Each of the enrolled fourteen couples was supplied with sixteen barrier devices and given both written and verbal instructions for their use, although three of the couples did not return for follow-up.

Initially, the researchers had hoped to recruit twenty to thirty volunteer couples, and the apparent lack of interest to participate in the study proved disappointing. Jobst and Johns speculated that:

> In further discussions with the study participants and among the clinic staff, it was felt that low interest to participate was attributed to lack of motivation among this group of couples. The perception among monogamous, HIV-antibody negative couples, with no incidence or perceived risk to AIDS or other STDs, is that there is no need to use any protective method. Further studies should consider modifying the study entrance criteria to motivate gay men who express interest to try a new device because they have a desire to use a protective device.[5]

The researchers drew attention to a key issue that is present in any study testing the effectiveness of an HIV-prevention device. Scientists are unable to ethically conduct an experiment on the efficacy of an unapproved barrier between HIV-positive and HIV-negative sex partners without risking the infection of their subjects for the purposes of data collection. For this reason, monogamous, HIV-negative couples were used to test Aegis for its durability, which was measured by the presence of leaks and tears. Unfortunately, because these couples did not need to use a barrier to prevent infection, the compliance of the research subjects was difficult to maintain throughout the course of the study.

Of the remaining eleven couples, a total of thirty-one devices were used during anal intercourse. Some of the condoms were retained by the couples after use and returned to the clinic for evaluation of possible breakage. In response to investigation of the first perspective of acceptability (breakage), one hundred percent of the returned Aegis barriers were free of any leaks or tears. As an overall alternative to the male latex condom, the Howard Brown researchers stated:

> All study participants found the conception of protection for the receptive partner acceptable. However, all responding participants found design and usage difficulties with the Aegis pouch. The design objectives were primarily related to feeling the seam and/or inner ring during intercourse.[6]

In the discussion and conclusion of the study, Jobst and Johns determined that more clearly emphasized instructions, additional lubricant, and gradual desensitization to the new and different design of such a barrier would alleviate the device's shortcomings.

SEXUAL GOVERNANCE

Despite the promising, albeit inconclusive, results of the Howard Brown clinic study, the FDA's eventual approval of the device in the United States came with numerous exclusions, including the exemption of language and directions for anal sex in all advertisements, promotional materials, and instructions enclosed in the packaged product. As a result, the restriction to vaginal use resulted in the Female Health Company changing the name of the device from "Aegis" to "Reality female condom." The FDA's reasoning for allegedly excluding anal-specific language in relation to Reality's marketing and use was justified by citing several states' sodomy laws, coupled with a resistance to "encourage" illegal behavior.

In recent years, the availability of medical technology has become increasingly mediated through government regulation and, simultaneously, the pleasures and protection of safer sex have been enhanced by emergent technology. The ease and ability to engage in specific forms of technologized safer sex have grown reliant upon the same institutions that have traditionally sought to systematically deter sexually deviant behavior, and it should come as no surprise that government approval of HIV-preventive devices are contingent upon adherence to the values of the "moral majority." Clearly, in the case of Reality, the politics of safer sex have become technologized and the technology of safer sex has become politicized.

A news article published by the *San Francisco Chronicle* explained, "Victor Zonana, a spokesman for the U.S. Department of Health and Human Services, which includes the FDA, acknowledged that previous administrations may have been reluctant to consider information related to use of such a device by gay men."[7] The previous administrations, of course, were the Republican administrations under Presidents Reagan and Bush. The *San Francisco Chronicle* also quoted Mary Ann Leeper, president of the Female Health Company, as stating, "I was told that anal intercourse is not approved in every state, so that I would not only have to fight battles related to the technology but also battles related to the politics of it."[8] The lack of the FDA's stamp of approval, however, is nothing unique. None of the traditional latex condoms on the market in the United States have been officially approved for anal use. Both latex condoms and Reality are approved for the prevention of pregnancy and sexually transmitted diseases, *but only for vaginal intercourse.*

Despite the FDA's prohibition in marketing and promoting Reality for anal use, gay men in the United States, Canada, and Europe have nonetheless begun to use the device as a safer-sex barrier method of preventing HIV transmission. England's *National AIDS Manual*, published in 1993, printed guidelines for Reality's use by gay men based on the Howard Brown Clinic study. Conspicuously, however, only a few mentionings of gay male usage of Reality appeared in newspapers, magazines, and other popular media before 1996. *POZ*, an HIV-lifestyle magazine, ran a story on Reality in late 1994, but only a few sentences of the article were devoted to the subject of gay men:

> We've heard there are gay men using it as well. The FDA sniffed at the topic: "We wouldn't have any opinion on male use of the [female] condom one way or the other." The marketer,

Female Health Company of Wisconsin Pharmacal, wasn't even surprised. "We support safer sex, period. Anyone who's having sex should do it safely and smartly, and here's one more option."[9]

An article titled, "A condom for her? We're curious . . ." ran on the front page of Canada's *Montreal Gazette* in January 1992. In the 1,318-word piece, one sentence buried in the middle mentions gay men. An unnamed representative of WPC was quoted as casually adding, "The female condom has been tested and found to be suitable for homosexual sex."[10] In his book *Safety in Numbers: Safer Sex and Gay Men*, Edward King makes brief mention of gay experimentation with the female condom. He quotes a piece in the December 1991 edition of the Toronto gay and lesbian periodical *Xtra!* that interviewed a local AIDS counselor about his personal experience with trying Reality.[11] Even as early as 1990, a *Boston Globe* article about the Sixth International Conference on AIDS mentioned an anonymous scientist who noted "that the 'female' condom might also reduce the risk of [HIV infection via] anal intercourse with *either* sex."[12] (Italics mine.)

So why would gay men choose to use an unapproved barrier device for anal sex rather than abide with conventional condoms? The comparative pros and cons between Reality and latex condoms are numerous. The advantages of Reality include the belief that there is sometimes more sexual control by the receptive (bottom) partner, who is usually more at risk for HIV infection. Because Reality is made of polyurethane, oil-based lubricants can be used that would ordinarily break down latex condoms, causing them to break. Due to stronger construction, there is less tearing, breakage, and slippage with Reality. In clinical trials of the device with heterosexual couples, the rip and tear rate was 0.2 percent, whereas the tear numbers for latex condoms are 14 percent.[13] Polyurethane also conducts heat better than latex, and Reality can be used by people who have allergies to latex and would be unable to use traditional condoms.

Additional advantages include the ability to insert Reality several hours before the anticipated sexual activity, or at least before the insertive partner becomes erect, resulting in an uninterrupted move from foreplay to penetrative sex. The protruding outer ring of the sheath covers more external surface of the body, possibly affording additional protection against some sexually transmitted diseases that are spread through skin-to-skin contact, such as syphilis, herpes, and genital warts. Because Reality clings to the body cavity rather than the penis, some insertive partners (tops) report greater freedom of movement and tactile sensation due to the increased friction between the penis and a barrier.

Perhaps the biggest disadvantage of Reality over latex condoms is cost, with the price of Reality being five to ten times more than the average latex condom. In terms of availability, latex condoms are more widely available for purchase in stores and distributed for free by many AIDS organizations and gay businesses. Other difficulties include the mechanics of insertion, for Reality is somewhat cumbersome and involves more complicated procedures and instructions for use. Some users, as evidenced by the Howard Brown Clinic study, have indicated they experience some discomfort related to feeling the inner ring and lengthwise seam of the sheath. Another reported complaint has been the noise of the device, that it makes "squishing" sounds as the lubricated plastic bunches up and crinkles. (This problem is easily solved with adding more lubricant.) Although some people may benefit from being able to use oil-based lubricants with the device, use of Reality cannot be followed with use of latex condoms, since these same oils will break down latex.

FEMINIZING SAFER SEX TECHNOLOGY

In a 1992 press release, U.S. manufacturer Wisconsin Pharmacal stated Reality was originally conceived for the benefit of women: "Reality was developed by a Danish physician who was concerned about transmission of STDs and felt that women needed a protective method to use themselves."[14] For a short time, Wisconsin Pharmacal and Howard Brown Clinic researchers considered the device to be a gender-neutral barrier pouch, although it was later reattributed specifically to women. This brief foray into gender neutrality and anal application signifies the key discursive movements when the device hesitantly approached gay male sexuality, then quickly distanced itself from the resulting political turbulence. It is important to recognize that the possibilities of anal reality were first explored by the manufacturer and clinicians associated with Reality, then later appropriated by gay men once they were denied official access to the product by the FDA.

Throughout Europe, the female condom bears the name "Femidom," a combination of the words feminine and condom. The sexual and gender implications of the female condom and its namesake are numerous and inescapable. That the word female has been added as a necessary descriptive adjective to condom indicates female entrance into a previously male domain. Even in labeling Reality a condom, rather than a barrier pouch as it was called during development studies, boundaries between male and female sexual technologies become blurred. During clinical testing the anticipated market name for the device had been Aegis, which has three general definitions: protection, sponsorship, or in Greek mythology, the shield or breastplate of Zeus, later an attribute of Athena, carrying at its center the head of Medusa. In North America, the symbolism of "Aegis" is rather significant. One might imagine allusions in the head of Medusa—phallic snakes, dangerous women with the ability to "harden" men, deadly desires, and so on. The device had previously possessed a kind of dual-gender personality, as with the protective gear of both Zeus and Athena.

Reality is marketed by a female (at least in name) business, the Female Health Company, and marketed to females, as the majority of Reality advertisements are found in publications such as *Cosmopolitan, Essence,* and *Mademoiselle,* aimed at predominantly heterosexual female audiences. The Reality logo consists of the text, "Reality female condom," circumscribed within a pink Venus female symbol (see Figure 2.1). Through this iconography, Reality becomes unavoidably and literally confined within a sphere of femaleness. In addition, it is marketed for female bodies. The box in which Reality is sold reads, "Reality is intended to be worn by women during sex." Due to FDA restrictions, the instruction booklet included in the packaging never even hints at the utility of Reality as an anal barrier, nor does it suggest use by men. The resultant feminization of the barrier pouch is no mistake. The very shifts in gendered nomenclature and marketing are indicative of the

FIGURE 2.1. Reality female condom Logo

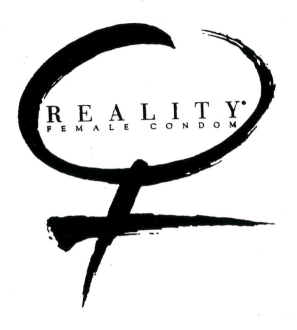

systems of heterosexism and erotophobia that government regulation employs in its policing of American sexuality. Even a statement issued by the FDA upon approval of Reality calls the device a "vaginal pouch" rather than a gender-neutral "barrier." [15]

The question of exactly who constitutes the user in the use of Reality is also significant and problematic. In virtually every instance, the Female Health Company defines the user of Reality to be female rather than male, as evidenced by the masthead text on the front of the box which reads, "An alternative for women." The wearer of the device translates into an equation with the user, even though within heterosexual use of Reality, the male partner *could* purchase, carry, initiate, and perform the insertion of the barrier. These actions are foregone, however, in the female user orientation of the device. Much of this orientation is situated within a justification for alternatives to latex condoms in the hopes of improving and sustaining safer sex behaviors. One of the chief complaints that heterosexual women have expressed over the last decade is that safer sex attempts are often discouraged, inhibited, or forcibly negated by their male partners. Gendered power inequities in heterosexual relations frequently subjugate women's attempts to protect themselves from HIV infection, and public health officials have declared a need for a female-controlled sexual barrier. Recognition of this problem is where the name Reality came from—a realistic look at some of the impediments to safer sex practices. In fact, a statement issued by the Department of Health and Human Services explained, "The agency [FDA] gave the product an expedited review because it saw an urgent need for a means whereby women can protect themselves without depending on the cooperation of their partners."[16]

Reality ambitiously claims to meet that need. Yet another statement on the box reads, "The alternative for women: take control of your health—use Reality." But what, exactly, makes Reality female-controlled? Other than the fact that the female is the wearer, social and cultural forces may still grant heterosexual men the power to remove the device or prevent its insertion by means of discouragement, manipulation, intimidation, and force. There is also a flawed assumption that it is, in every case, the insertive partner who is reluctant to use condoms, when sometimes it may be the receptive partner, or both partners who share this reluctance. This supposition has carried over into discussions of gay men who practice receptive anal intercourse, touted as an advantage for gay male appropriation of Reality.

INSTRUCTING THE ANUS

The totality of the packaged Reality, including the device(s), lubricant, and instructions, belie the attempt to inextricably confine it to contraception and female reproductive health. Even the illustrated diagrams depict only female bodies—as if to render the possibility of anal insertion visually unimaginable. The final version of the instructions enclosed with Reality are different from those provided to gay male couples in the Howard Brown Clinic study. The process of conducting the 1991 clinical study with gay male participants necessitated the design of gay-specific textual instructions accompanied by male anatomical diagrams and illustrations (Figures 2.2 and 2.3). Interestingly, the 1991 Aegis instructions address a wide range of sexual behaviors beyond penis-to-anus intercourse. A question and answer portion of the booklet even included the following queries:

Q: Can Aegis be used for fisting?
A: No. Aegis is designed for penile insertion only.

Q: Can Aegis be used in water sports activities?
A: No. Aegis is not designed for activities involving urine.

Q: Can Aegis be used in oral/anal sex?
A: Yes, providing the outer ring remains outside the anus and all contact is protected by the barrier sheath.[17]

There appear to be some built-in assumptions about gay male sexuality here, as compared to the heterosexually sanitized instruction booklet that is commercially packaged with Reality. Although the answers to questions about use of Reality for water sports and fisting are a definitive "no," even the implication that people engage in these practices seems too risqué for user guidelines marketed to the public. Language pertaining to penis-to-anus intercourse is of course noticeably absent in the final Reality product, but the omission of guidance related to questions of fisting, water sports, and analingus is also significant. This demonstrates that Reality's utility has narrowed not only to the exclusion of anal intercourse, but all other conceivable forms of adapted sexual employment as well. The gaps in Reality's instructions speak volumes to the discomfort and apprehension associated with sexual behaviors that deviate from heterosexual, penis-to-vagina penetration.

The above activities (fisting, analingus, water sports) are not physically limited to an engagement between male bodies. Heterosexuals and lesbian women can and do participate in these activities. Especially where the rectum is concerned, however, a lack of gender-specificity in anatomical reference incites a particular heterosexual

FIGURE 2.2. Aegis Barrier Pouch—Instructions for Use

Aegis Barrier Pouch

QUESTIONS YOU MAY HAVE

1 What do I do if the outer ring is pushed inside when the penis enters?

STOP. Remove *Aegis* and insert again according to these directions. Put extra lubricant at the opening of the anus. We suggest lubricating the insertive penis before you begin to put *Aegis* back in.

2 Why would the outer ring go inside?

As you know, we all have different anatomical sizes. In some cases, the amount of lubricant in *Aegis* may not be enough. If the outer ring does go inside, remove *Aegis* and add extra lubricant at the opening of the anus before putting it back in.

3 Will *Aegis* bunch up inside?

Aegis should not bunch up inside if it is inserted right and if there is enough lubricant in the sheath. If either you or your partner notices the outer ring begin to slip inside, **STOP.** Pull the outer ring to lie outside the anus as in fig. H. Add extra lubricant.

4 What do I do if the penis is inserted outside the outer ring?

STOP. Remove penis. Be sure the outer ring lies flat over the anal area.

5 Will *Aegis* rip or tear while I am using it?

Studies show that it is unlikely for *Aegis* to **rip or tear during use. If this does occur, remove it right away, throw it away, and insert a new *Aegis*.**

INVESTIGATIONAL DEVICE NOT
AEGIS
The Female
Chicago /
1-800-

REGARDING THE PROPER USE

6 **Is *Aegis* too short?**

No. *Aegis* has been designed to fit the aver-aged size penis.

7 **Should I or my partner wear a conventional condom while using *Aegis* for anal sex?**

It is not necessary because in effect *Aegis* is a condom, covering the penis and the anal cavity during sex.

8 **Can *Aegis* be used for fisting?**

No. *Aegis* is designed for penile insertion only.

9 **Can *Aegis* be used in oral/anal sex?**

Yes, providing the outer ring remains outside the anus and all contact is protected by the barrier sheath.

10 **Can *Aegis* be used in watersports activities?**

No. *Aegis* is not designed for activities involving urine.

Notes:

If used properly:

- Latex condoms for men are highly effective at preventing sexually transmitted diseases, including AIDS (HIV).
- If you are not going to use a male latex condom, you can use the *Aegis* to help protect yourself and your partner.
- Withdrawing before climax (before coming) will further reduce the risk.

APPROVED FOR MARKETING

Health Company
London
274-6601

FIGURE 2.3. Aegis Barrier Pouch—Instructions for Use

Aegis   INSTRUCTIONS

Barrier Pouch   NOTE: *Aegis* is an INVESTIGATIONAL

1   Some important points to know

1. *Aegis* gives the Receptive Partner a way to protect himself. It can be inserted any time prior to sex. It warms up on insertion.
2. The polyurethane material used in the *Aegis* sheath is stronger than the latex used in conventional condoms, yet it is soft.
3. *Aegis* gives broader protection because it covers the outer area of the anus and the base of the penis during anal sex.
4. *Aegis* <u>does not</u> deteriorate when oil-based lubricants are used.

4

- Take out *Aegis* and look at it closely.
- Be sure the lubrication is evenly spread inside the pouch from the bottom to the top by rubbing the outside of the pouch together.
- If you need to, add more lubricant. Simply give one quick squeeze of the extra lubricant provided. You can decide how much more you and your partner would like once you try it. You can also use oil-based lubricants.

2   Don't tear *Aegis*   *fig. A*

Be careful of sharp objects, like rings or sharp fingernails.

Outer Ring

Aegis Barrier Pouch

Inner Ring

5   To insert *Aegis*   *fig. C*

- Be sure the **inner-ring is at the bottom, closed-end** of the pouch.
- If you wish, **add** extra lubricant to the outside of the pouch for extra comfort when you insert *Aegis.*

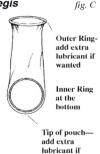

Outer Ring— add extra lubricant if wanted

Inner Ring at the bottom

Tip of pouch— add extra lubricant if wanted.

3   Practice putting *Aegis* in before you plan to actually use it   *fig. B*

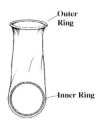

- Get familiar with *Aegis's* unusual shape and looks.
- See how it hangs outside of the anus when in place, lining the anal cavity.
- Make sure you are comfortable inserting *Aegis* <u>before</u> you use it in sex.

6   How to hold the sheath   *fig. D*

- Hold the inner ring between thumb and middle finger. Put index finger on pouch between other two fingers, (or)
- Just squeeze.

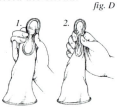
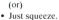

FOR USE

DEVICE limited by Federal Law to investigational use.

7

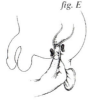

fig. E

- Still squeezing *Aegis* with your fingers, insert the device through the anal opening as shown in fig. E. Take your time. If *Aegis* is slippery to insert, let go and start over.

The inner ring helps insert Aegis. It also helps to hold it in place during sex.

8

fig. F

- Now push the inner ring and the pouch the rest of the way up into the anal cavity with your index finger.
- For maximum protection, the inner ring should be inserted past the sphincter muscle. See fig. F.
- This step may be hard to do on the first or second try.

9 | Before Anal Sex

fig. G

- When you are ready for sex, insert *Aegis*, making sure the outside ring lies outside the anus as shown in fig. G.
- About one inch of the open end will stay outside. See fig. H. While this may look unusual, this part of *Aegis* is protecting you and your partner during sex.
- You can add more lubricant either inside or outside *Aegis* for extra comfort.

Outside ring correctly outside Aegis.

10 | During Anal Sex

fig. H

You may notice that *Aegis* moves around during sex.
- Moving side-to-side of the outer ring is **normal.** It will not reduce your protection.
- Sometimes *Aegis* may slip up and down in the anal cavity, riding on the penis. However the penis should remain **covered** by the pouch and any fluid stays inside the pouch.
- **But, if** either you or your partner notice the outer ring being pushed into the anal cavity, **STOP.** Pull the outer ring so that it lies outside the anus and add extra lubricant to the opening of the pouch or to the insertive penis. Make sure the outer ring lies outside the anus.
- If the penis starts to enter underneath or beside the sheath, **STOP** and reinsert within the covered anus.

10 | During Anal Sex

fig. I

To take out *Aegis*, **squeeze and twist the outer ring** to keep any fluid inside the pouch. **Pull out** gently. Throw away in a trash can. **DO NOT FLUSH. DO NOT REUSE.**

Twisting holds the seminal fluid inside the pouch.

panic, inasmuch as the anus eludes a stable categorization. In her book *Inventing AIDS*, cultural theorist Cindy Patton discusses the hetero's denial of anal pleasure and the anus's deeply disturbing "lack of gender reference. Thus, desires centering on the anus cannot infallibly be stabilized to produce 'heterosexuality,' and anal sex becomes a key site of (hetero)sexual danger through loss of gender reference."[18] The relegation of anal sex to an activity that takes place only between gay men shores up this distress, for it not only queers the anus, but gender specifies it as a cavity of inherently male pleasure. When it comes to an internal condom, the key difference between the vagina and anus becomes one of gender. The female condom thus becomes equated with vaginal use through the gender-specification of this sexual technology's user. Denial of heterosexual anal intercourse seems to be enough to presume that consumers would never use Reality for anything other than its marketed purpose.

However, open promotion of the female condom as being functional for anal practices has created a rough terrain that is fraught with heterosexual anxiety. This becomes especially evident in the FDA's alleged refusal of Reality to be marketed as an anal appliance based on state sodomy laws. While these anxieties might be calmed and comforted through the discursive silences and omissions of male homosexuality and anal pleasure, gay men are literally left to their own devices when it comes to safer sex options. There continues to be a lack of instruments specifically designed, researched, and approved for safer anal intercourse, symptomatic of a more general neglect of gay male sexual health and wellness.

QUEERING REALITY

So what does all this gender specifying and heterosexualizing of Reality (and reality) mean for gay men who might consider using the device? In order to begin sketching out the many factors that play into this, I conducted an informal survey in 1997 on the Internet of gay men who have used Reality at least once. One of the respondents, who simply calls himself Joe, pointed me to his World Wide Web site dedicated to Reality. Joe, who lives in Amsterdam, has used the female condom exclusively for over two years now. He is so pleased with the device, in fact, that he has written an article titled "Sexual Engineering," found at his Web site. The informal interviews, Joe's electronic article, print media, and a consumer survey conducted by a San Francisco AIDS organization informed my attempt to discern, at least anecdotally, the hows and whys of gay men's Reality.

For some, the appropriation of female condoms is even accompanied by a suggested name change to designate receptive or passive sexual roles rather than biological sex of the receptive sexual partner. Joe, for example, proclaims, "The user-friendly condom has arrived, in the form of the 'female condom'—what could properly be called the 'bottom' condom, an engineering triumph for all of us . . ."[19] Beyond the nicknames that Reality has acquired in its appropriation for anal sex, the queer adaptation of it has carved out a wide range of new and renewed sexual possibilities for men who have sex with men, detailed below.

Foreplay

An article published in the gay male leather magazine *Drummer* indicates insertion of Reality may serve as actual preparation, beyond protection, for anal sex by relaxing the sphincter muscles: ". . . whereas many men find the process of putting a condom on the top disruptive, the insertion of the Reality condom can readily become part of the top's ritual of loosening the bottom for penetration."[20] In e-mail correspondence, Joe told me "I put it on (in) basically the same way, except of course I have no cervix to fit it over. It is also highly entertaining to play with someone's asshole with lubricant, and slide it in, etc. as opposed to rolling on a rubber."[21]

Early Insertion

The London newspaper *The Observer* reported, "One health care worker in a London hospital said a patient who had never used condoms in the past was using the Femidom: 'He inserts it before going cruising and does not have to ask whoever he has sex with to wear a condom.'"[22] In Philadelphia, the Gay and Latino AIDS Education organization operates a program called Midnight Cowboy that conducts safer sex outreach to male sex workers. Hassan J.

Gibbs of Midnight Cowboy explained to the *Philadelphia Inquirer* that male sex workers were beginning to use Reality for anal sex in part because of the ability to insert the device in advance. Joe reports from Amsterdam, with tongue in cheek, that he "imagines that people could put one in and go out for the evening pre-prepared for spontaneous safer sex in terribly irresponsible situations, but again this would only be appropriate for strict scientific evaluation of this product. Or something like that . . . Have fun in research!" Quite consciously, Joe points to the inevitable tensions between scientific enabling and moral disapproval of casual sex with anonymous or multiple partners, for the only continued research on gay male use of Reality is occurring at this kind of grass-roots level.

Analingus

Reality has been touted as an effective barrier for oral-anal contact (rimming) by *Drummer,* a gay men's magazine as well as the Howard Brown clinic investigators. An article published in *Drummer,* a periodical geared toward the gay male leather and S/M communities, points out that Reality can be used for analingus, stating that "The condom also protects against passage of cryptosporidium and parasites during rimming."[23]

Duration

In Joe's World Wide Web home page, he discusses how the female condom might actually enable and prolong anal sex:

> Unless you are particularly fond of the sometimes unpleasant friction on your asshole while being fucked, there is none of the tugging and tearing that you get even with well-lubricated ordinary condoms. What used to be uncomfortable after ten minutes will now last indefinitely.[24]

Oil-Based Lubricants

A reminiscence or return to pre-AIDS sexual behavior may also provide a degree of appeal to some gay men. Joe indicated that the small bottle of lubricant included with the condom "felt like mineral oil or baby oil (yes, it may be time for Crisco again!)"[25] For Joe, being able to use an oil-based lubricant once again, even with a barrier, signifies a certain pleasure in returning to the 1970s, a time when Crisco and Vaseline were widely popular for use with anal sex in gay male communities. Echoing this nostalgia, San Francisco AIDS activist Michael Petrelis stated that using Reality is "like having sex in the 70s again."[26] The first-edition of *The Joy of Gay Sex*, published in 1977, declared, "Vegetable shortening may be the best lubricant, since it is not only greasy but also digestible."[27] In the 1978 sex manual *The Advocate Guide to Gay Health*, Crisco even earned an entry in the book's index. Discussions of the short-ening's use as an anal lubricant indicate its popularity, with state-ments such as: "The lubricant, typically the cultic Crisco, must be copious."[28] Given that such oil-based substances break down or-dinary latex condoms and cause them to break, this new option holds understandable appeal for men who had standardly used oils in the past and discontinued them with the adoption of safer sex practices. In addition, younger gay men may find the possibility of safer experimentation with oil-based lubricants appealing. The polyurethane material of newly developed safer sex technologies may grant them an opportunity to partake in sexual activities their older gay counterparts previously enjoyed but they themselves have been denied with the early 1980s advent of AIDS.

Sensation

In e-mail correspondence, one anonymous gay man told me that, "since it does not fit rigidly on the penis like the traditional con-doms do, there is greater sensitivity to the penis. . . . It [the condom] stays in one place and the penis has greater tactile responses." Joe reports that, "Probably the nicest part of it all is the feeling—once the condom is in place in the ass, you absolutely don't notice it." Another gay male fan of Reality recounted, "When I was doing the fucking, I did notice the interior ring a bit at first, until it got pushed out of the way. But in terms of sensation, it was great. When I was being fucked, it didn't feel as if there was a device in me at all."[29] Hassan J. Gibbs of Philadelphia's Midnight Cowboy program told the *Philadelphia Inquirer* that male sex workers use Reality, "And if it's dark enough, the johns never even know."[30]

Other Uses

Continuing to espouse the advantages of the female condom, Joe suggests reusing part of the prophylactic after the initial act of anal sex: "The inner ring makes a nice invisible cockring, by the way." The flexibility, diameter, and opacity of the inner ring lends itself to later use as a sexual device which, when placed tightly around the base of the penis and testicles, constricts blood flow. The reduced circulation traps blood in the penis, maintaining extended periods of erection and prolonging ejaculation. Steven Gibson, Community Organizer of the STOP AIDS Project in San Francisco, reported that the local gay male leather community seems to have taken a particular liking to Reality due to its polyurethane design. He suggested that the plastic composition makes it erotically appealing for those who possess a fetish for plastic clothing and sex toys. In addition to these new applications, the fact that Reality may actually make anal sex physically easier and more possible than ever before transforms the device into an appliance of moral danger, a modern convenience of sexual perversity in contemporary Western culture.

On December 1, 1996, the STOP AIDS Project began distributing 500 Reality condoms to gay men throughout San Francisco, asking them to use the devices for anal sex, complete an accompanying consumer survey of their experience, and return the information to the organization. The study was coordinated by Steven Gibson and the San Francisco Department of Public Health AIDS Office donated the condoms and conducted the data analysis. One hundred of the surveys were returned. The data that were collected offered some promise of users' acceptability of the alternative barrier device. Preliminary results stated, "Approval for using the Reality condom was very high. Eighty-six percent of the respondents said they would use the condom again. Fifty-four percent said they would rather use the Reality condom than a conventional condom." As for complications with use of Reality for anal sex, gay men reported, "Obstacles included cost ($10 for a 3 pack), possible misuse, appearance and interest may drop off as its novelty dissipates."[31]

STOP AIDS publicized the results of the study by hosting a community forum on anal sex in August of 1997. The local gay and lesbian community newspaper, *Bay Area Reporter*, enumerated some of the more detailed findings. "Another key finding of the survey was that men who are not in monogamous relationships rated the Reality condom significantly higher than men in monogamous relationships. For men in monogamous relationships, the approval rating for the anal condom was higher among serodiscordant couples; these couples also reported they are more likely to use the condom again."[32] STOP AIDS's draft summary of the survey concluded, "The fact that a large proportion of men in the study preferred the Reality condom over conventional condoms may increase consistent condom use for anal sex. There still is no magic bullet to stop HIV transmission. Prevention is our best answer. The Reality condom provides another option for gay and bisexual men."[33]

As for continued research in this area, two additional studies have been conducted that merit attention. A survey of more than 2,000 HIV-negative gay men in six different U.S. cities (Boston, Chicago, Denver, New York, San Francisco, and Seattle) practicing anal sex, found 148 (7 percent of the total cohort) had used Reality within the previous six months, with highest rates of use in San Francisco and Seattle.[34] Researchers also gathered data on problems with the device, likelihood of future use, and more.

More concrete information on Reality's effectiveness for anal sex may ultimately come from outside the United States, however. A group of gay men's health organizations in the United Kingdom have banded together to conduct research in this area and, unlike the United States, have formal ties to Chartex International—the international manufacturer of Reality (or Femidom, as it is called in Europe). Douglas T. Newberry of the Salisbury Gay Men's Health Project predicts, "If Femidom is proven to be safe, Chartex would consider an alternative marketing strategy to attract gay men to the product."[35] It remains to be seen whether or not this alternative would influence the FDA's rigid restrictions in the United States.[35]

THE SAN FRANCISCO CONTROVERSY

In 1996, San Francisco AIDS activist Michael Petrelis visited a sex shop called Good Vibrations, where he learned of gay men's use of the female condom for anal sex. He decided to try the condom with his male partner, and liked it so much that he launched a campaign to spread the word about Reality's benefits. He also became enraged that the city health department was not promoting it for anal use and that San Francisco public health clinics were only distributing female condoms to women as part of their free provision of safer sex materials throughout the city. He pressured the San Francisco City AIDS Office with a barrage of phone calls and memos, and created a publicity buzz by distributing press releases to local and national media demanding that the condom be made widely available to gay men for anal intercourse.

Soon thereafter, in March of 1996, San Francisco AIDS Office Director Mitch Katz issued a memo instituting a policy to distribute female condoms to gay men at the city's health clinics. In the memo addressed to district health center directors, Katz stated: "The position of the Department is that we recommend the use of regular condoms for anal sex. Clients need to know that Reality female condoms are not approved by the FDA for this use, but it is our intention to make them available, especially for clients unwilling to use regular condoms."[36] Katz couched this decision in language which conveyed that the health department would offer Reality to gay men who are otherwise noncompliant with safer sex guidelines, providing them with an unusual and untested substitute rather than leave them completely unprotected. In part, the decided risk of providing an inadequately tested barrier shifts any liability to gay men who are unwilling to use regular condoms. The policy was justified as more of a last-ditch emergency effort to reach supposedly uncooperative gay men, rather than stating that Reality may be a device which many gay men prefer over latex condoms for very valid material and cultural reasons.

A quantity of 500 Reality condoms were purchased for distribution, and the health department took the anal-specific instruction booklet from the Howard Brown Clinic study and refashioned it into a double-sided flyer to be given out along with them. The flyer also includes the following disclaimer:

> Warning: The Reality condom has not been tested as a barrier against HIV infection. The Reality condom is not approved by the FDA for anal intercourse. The San Francisco Department of Public Health recommends using a latex penile condom for

anal sex. However, we want to make anal condoms available for use by men because we recognize some men may prefer anal condoms, and we believe that it is better to use an anal condom than none at all.[37]

The difference between the language used by the San Francisco health department in the official memo and their language used for direct communication to gay men is subtle, but apparent. The health department states in its memorandum that distribution of Reality is in response to gay men who are unwilling to use regular condoms, whereas the instructional flyer softens this statement by communicating an attempt to meet some gay men's prefer[ence] for Reality. The flyer also carefully avoids ever calling Reality a female condom, relying on other terms such as Reality condom, device, pouch, and more important, anal condom. Through these linguistic maneuvers, the confusion of female condom use for gay male sex is conveniently sidestepped.

This decision to disseminate Reality for anal sex in San Francisco attracted a great deal of media attention, largely due to the press releases and media advocacy conducted by Petrelis, who demanded attention to the issue and publicly condemned the FDA for not approving an anal Reality. The local San Francisco media, Associated Press, and national gay press picked up the story instantly. Petrelis also took out a full page ad in the Washington, DC, gay newspaper, *The Washington Blade*, reprinting the *Bay Area Reporter*'s front page feature titled "FDA Denies Reality to Gays." Several newspapers reprinted the medical illustration of Reality being inserted into the rectum. For the first time, a visual depiction of an anal Reality was disseminated to hundreds of thousands of people. In the name of journalism and reporting on current affairs, do-it-yourself instructions for appropriation of Reality were offered on a mass scale to anyone who might be interested.

Gay journalist Gabriel Rotello dedicated a full page opinion column to the subject in the national gay and lesbian news magazine, *The Advocate*, in which he asked, "How would you feel if you found out that years ago researchers created a product with the potential to slash the HIV infection rate among gay men—but were told by the federal government to forget about it?"[38] Although

Reality had been denied to gay men for years, actively by the FDA and passively through the Female Health Company's discursive silences in marketing, Petrelis was able to imbue the dispute with a sense of urgency needed to create public conversation and at least limited action. That summer at the Eleventh International Conference on AIDS, Petrelis even organized a "Kiss-In for Anal Rights" demonstration at the Female Health Company's booth in the exhibit hall of the conference site.

Most gay men in San Francisco certainly seem to be aware of Reality's appropriation. Safer sex product vendors in the city such as Mercury Mail Order, Condomania, and others report they sell so many female condoms to gay men that they "can't keep them on the shelves." The Walgreen's Pharmacy at the corner of 18th and Castro Streets in the gay ghetto of San Francisco report selling large quantities of Reality to gay customers, although they are unable to quantify the consumer demographics of these sales. The significance of pharmacy sales include the numbers of gay men who obtain Reality by prescription from their physician. In their reporting of the controversies surrounding Reality, the *Bay Area Reporter* worked subversively to spread the word that Californians can receive reimbursement for their Reality purchase from the state government if they qualify for MediCal and can find a physician who is willing to write a prescription for the device. The article even cited the billing, product, and manufacturer codes that physicians need to complete the paperwork.[39] Ironically, while the federal government has refused to sanction an anal Reality, the state of California is subsidizing many gay men's purchase of Reality for anal sex through state Medicare programs.

San Francisco's precedent has not set off a chain reaction of similar implementation in other city health departments, however. Marcy Fraser of the San Francisco City AIDS Office reported that while several gay men contacted her amidst the media hype to inquire about anal use of Reality, she received only one call from any other health organization—the Seattle health department.[40]

But now there are media reports of Reality distribution to gay men in Philadelphia and Chicago as well. Carol Rogers of the Philadelphia Department of Public Health told the Associated Press that distribution of Reality to gay men has been met with success.

"We've had a lot of response from men who have sex with men and they like it very much."[41] Response to Reality distribution seems, by and large, quite favorable, but health departments nationwide have not demonstrated any particular eagerness to initiate their own programs.

THE APPROPRIATENESS OF APPROPRIATION

Not everyone agrees that gay men should be appropriating Reality for anal intercourse, however. In 1993 Peter Tatchell, a founding member of ACT UP London, described gay men as "sexual magpies who adapt all kinds of inventions to fulfill their desire for erotic innovation."[42] The term "magpie," when applied to humans rather than birds, refers to someone who "collects or hoards things, especially indiscriminately."[43] This curious word choice provides analogies between promiscuity and hoarding, and casual sex with indiscrimination, diminishing use of Reality as simply the latest trend in gay men's excessive orgasmic pursuit. Tatchell has refused to recommend the female condom in his new AIDS-prevention guidebook unless the device is improved. He feels there is a need and a market for a prophylactic device "designed specifically for anal sex."[44]

Taking a similar stance, Ben Schatz, member of the Presidential Advisory Council on AIDS and executive director of the Gay and Lesbian Medical Association, has argued that actively encouraging gay men to use the Reality condom without more testing of the device's efficacy would be irresponsible.[45]

There is also the question of prohibitive cost and gender-specific allocation of AIDS-prevention resources. Currently, Reality condoms cost $1.66 each if purchased in bulk. The cost of latex condoms purchased in bulk directly from manufacturers ranges from six to thirty cents apiece. (Over the counter, latex condoms cost approximately sixty cents apiece and Reality costs around three dollars apiece.) Many public health officials and AIDS-prevention workers question whether mass distribution of Reality is the best use of limited dollars in waging the war against new infections.

In addition, many organizations are purchasing female condoms with funds from their women's health budget and then distributing them to men who have sex with men. What does this mean for tenuous relationships within communities competing for resources and attempting to work in collaboration for an integrated approach to reducing rates of infection? Marcy Fraser of the San Francisco Health Department has noted that, "There is some concern from women that with our limited resources and supplies, this could put a crimp in the supply (of condoms) for women . . . We just don't have enough money."[46] Lauri Irving, aide to Supervisor Tom Amimiano of the San Francisco Health Department, told the *Bay Area Reporter*, "I'm all for passing them out if they save lives . . . but I worry about diverting funds from women and not replacing them. We should focus on expanding resources."[47] These concerns were exacerbated by Michael Petrelis's appeal to the San Francisco Human Rights Commission, which included charges that the denied distribution of Reality to gay men constituted sex discrimination. Petrelis did not, however, acknowledge or advocate for heterosexual women's anal use of Reality. Robin Gorna, Head of Health Promotion at Terrence Higgins Trust in England, has been one of the few individuals to even mention heterosexual women's use of the female condom for anal sex. In the conclusion of her book, *Vamps, Virgins, and Victims: How Can Women Fight AIDS?*, Gorna maps out an agenda for women to fight AIDS on numerous fronts, including the advisement that we should "Promote the delights of female condoms as well as their problems! Campaign for the development of a wide range of protection mechanisms (e.g., polyurethane condoms), and ensure they are tested for anal sex as well as vaginal sex."[48]

As for the government opposition to approval of an anal barrier device, the future of Reality will be at least somewhat dependent on federal partisan politics. The FDA, now operating under a much more liberal and gay-friendly Presidential administration, has publicly stated they are willing to discuss and consider approval for anal marketing of Reality. Mitch Katz of the San Francisco Health Department has stated that,

> The product is not approved for this [anal] use by the FDA. The company that manufactures "Reality" did a very limited study five years ago on its use as an anal condom. The results were taken to the FDA who, at that time, did not consider

them. This position may have been based on conservative sexual mores. It is our understanding that they are now willing to revisit that decision.[49]

The Female Health Company, however, has failed to seek this approval under the Clinton presidential administration or begin these discussions. Nor do they plan to do so in the foreseeable future, according to their marketing salesperson Holly Birnbaum Sherman. She cites a continuing fear that, should the Female Health Company seek anal approval, the product will be pulled from the market altogether. However, even if the FDA is willing to grant this approval, it is neither the responsibility nor the function of the government agency to initiate this approval process with a privately owned, profit-driven company. The status of official approval of Reality for anal use is caught up in a stalemate of inaction, and no one seems quite sure who to hold responsible. The FDA could be feigning gay and anal friendliness, misrepresenting their intentions to avoid outraged activism from the gay community and resultant negative publicity; and the financially struggling Female Health Company may not want to officially endorse their product for anal use, as this could stigmatize Reality as a gay condom and sour their largely heterosexual female clientele. Ben Schatz told the *Bay Area Reporter* that, "Every indication I've gotten from HHS [Health and Human Services] is that they're open to the concept of testing internal condoms for anal usage. . . . Once the FDA is open, then it's up to the manufacturer. Many of us want to see research done on its applicability and effectiveness for anal use, but you can't force a manufacturer to test a product."[50]

Reactions from conservative Christian organizations were also swift and harsh once the media began to report the anal potential of Reality. Mike Russell, a spokesperson for the Christian Coalition, told the Associated Press, "It would be our view that the government would have a very tough time approving such a product. They are promoting an activity that is clearly illegal in more than twenty states."[51] The Christian Coalition's statement appears to be one of mere reactionary opinion rather than active campaigning, for they have articulated neither a grass-roots appeal nor a legislative agenda concerning anal condoms. Their threat remains significant, however, in that it represents the possibility for formidable opposition from an organized social movement. Female Health Company Mary Ann Leeper also told the Associated Press that anal approval of Reality would be "a political basketball that's going to be batted around . . . We're too small. We couldn't survive that."[52]

The *Bay Area Reporter* stated that, "According to Richard Sorian, a press representative in the office of national AIDS Czar Patsy Fleming, after the panel's statement was reported in the B.A.R., his boss 'made inquiries to the FDA and the Department of Health and Human Services,' and they are being pursued."[53] The results of these inquiries have never been communicated to the public. In fact, no one can quote the FDA's alleged 1991 communication that anal inclusion of Reality would result in a total rejection of the device altogether. Only off-the-record conversations are recounted. There do not seem to be transcripts of these statements excluding anal use. Some have reported the FDA blatantly refused to consider Reality for anal use, while Dr. Lillian Yin, who was head of the FDA at the time, told the *Bay Area Reporter* that the results of the Aegis study were "never brought in for approval."[54]

One must also wonder, in this cast of individual and organizational actors, where gay community leadership stands amidst these controversies? Neither the National Lesbian and Gay Health Association nor the Gay and Lesbian Medical Association have made a formal organizational statement or taken a stance on the issue of gay men's anal appropriation of Reality. A disturbing contradiction becomes apparent in this silence, evidenced by an eager willingness to advocate for new HIV treatments, even untested and dangerous ones, yet there has been no consistent effort to push for new HIV *preventions*. In her discussion of the female condom, Robin Gorna has noted that, "In the midst of a crisis which is so complex and changing, perhaps the certainty of a central prevention method gives reassurance and stability."[55] The introduction of new safer sex technologies heaps a greater burden upon AIDS educators, public health officials, and sexually active individuals. In the mid-1980s, the classic instruction of "use a condom, every time" was presumed to be a sufficient response to safer sex inquiries. In the late 1990s, however, such questions as "Which protection is best for which kind of penetration with which kind of lubricant and which kind of partner?" have arisen from newly available internal condoms and polyurethane penile condoms. This comes in addition to the complexities of protease inhibitor and other drug treatments; viral load testing and other surrogate markers for assessing HIV disease; changes in public policy and legal precedent; and the development of oral and urinary HIV-antibody tests. Educating the public about AIDS has become a near-impossible job in a time of rapid change, and the simplicity of traditional latex condoms may win out over technologies that, while possessing certain advantages, require more time and money to disseminate with proper instructions.

Whatever the reasons for continued absence of approval for Reality as an anal device, the so-called female condom is the latest site where gay male sexuality is regulated, scrutinized, negotiated, and technologized. In response to this lack of approval, gay men's appropriation of female-specific safer sex technology reveals a need for newly engineered devices that take advantage of recent technological advances that can make sexual practices safer and more pleasurable than ever before. In 1997, the medical journal *Sexually Transmitted Diseases* published "Use and Effectiveness of Condoms During Anal Intercourse: A Review" by Barbara Silverman and Thomas Gross, both of the Center for Devices and Radiological Health in the Food and Drug Administration.

> Increasing the effectiveness of condoms, particularly for anal use, will require development of new devices that resist slippage and breakage and present less of a challenge for the inexperienced user. Although there is some evidence to suggest that it is possible to engineer a condom to better withstand the stresses of anal intercourse, such a product may be rejected by many users as a result of comfort and sensation.[56]

Silverman and Gross fail to make mention of the female condom anywhere in their extensive review, and suggest the engineering of a better condom for anal sex would be beneficial. They fail to acknowledge, however, that such a device already exists and is being used by gay men around the world. This form of denial, especially when emanating from within the same federal agency that denied anal approval of Reality, is symptomatic of an imaginary world where the development, naming, marketing, consumption, and use of Reality are all possessed of the utmost irony, especially if we consider the opposite of reality to be the imaginary.

Despite the encouraging conclusions reached by the Howard Brown Clinic study, no further clinical research of Reality's potential for anal use has been conducted. While public health officials and government regulation agencies continue to debate the appropriateness, legality, and effectiveness of a rectal Reality, gay men and others who practice anal sex are left with one less option to protect themselves amidst the ongoing AIDS pandemic. Further study of Reality's efficacy with anal sexual practices is crucial, as is a comprehensive plan to design and disseminate a broad range of technologies that create more opportunities for gay men to have sex, in all its forms, safely.

Threadbare Back

On the street outside Spin Cycle
I found him willing to interrupt
his load for me, so weighted
with twin duffles of spun
soaked cloth we set
out to the closer of our two places.

I was willing to bear half
his burden but he observed,
"The balance of two
makes the carry okay."
I smiled while sensing
something between us.

Face down on fresh sheets of threads
woven tight as the moment,
I considered how men were not
supposed to touch unsheathed.
His hips struck mine in gentle cycles,
powerful rhythms of closeness
that dampened my back.

Underneath I tried not to imagine
the pepper of mildew across
wet fabric waiting,
because I wanted to join him,
enjoy him, join with him,
with nothing between us.

Chapter 3

Condomless Condoms:
The Politics and Prospects
of Rectal Microbicides

At 1996's Eleventh International Conference on AIDS in Vancouver, the Clinton administration pledged 100 million dollars toward the development of topical agents for application prior to sexual activity that would reduce the risk of HIV infection. These protective creams or gels, known as microbicides, would ideally inactivate harmful bacteria, virus, and other microbes. The difficulty of developing a microbicide for internal use that would be hostile to dangerous pathogens while harmless to the user has been discussed for well over a decade. Early versions of contraceptive microbicides in the form of spermicidal films, foams, and jellies have been available for nearly twenty years in a variety of over-the-counter and prescription pharmaceutical products. More recently, however, a sense of urgency in the face of the AIDS pandemic has generated renewed interest in these chemical barriers.

The vast majority of discussion, research, and monetary commitment in developing microbicides has been directed toward products for vaginal use. Similar to the female condom, public health officials have repeatedly called for a safer sex technology that could be truly female controlled. In contrast to the female condom, vaginal microbicides could be used by women without her male sexual partner's knowledge. A potential ingredient for development of this kind of product is a substance called nonoxynol-9 (N-9), which has shown promise as both a spermicide and viricide when used internally. N-9 works by disrupting the cell membranes of microbes until they cannot survive, but studies of N-9 have generated mixed results, especially in evaluation of the substance as a prophylaxis to HIV infection. Despite the lack of conclusive evidence pertaining to the effectiveness of N-9 in reducing the risk of HIV transmission, several manufacturers of other popular sexual lubricants (e.g., Wet and ForePlay) have nonetheless included small amounts in their products with prominent labeling, suggesting that N-9 grants some additional amount of protection.

Perhaps the deepest concern regarding the use of N-9 resulted from the findings of a 1992 study conducted on Kenyan sex workers in which frequent use of the microbicide, delivered by an inserted sponge, seemed to cause a threefold increase in vaginal ulceration.[1] Rather than affording a heightened level of protection from infection, the irritation and resultant tissue damage could actually increase susceptibility by allowing pathogens greater penetration of the mucosa to reach the bloodstream. An inability to regulate the concentration of N-9 once applied internally has consistently discouraged researchers in their quest to design a product that would sustain a timely duration of protection in a nontoxic concentration.

In 1997, however, Columbia Labs Inc. in Miami, Florida, announced they had secured a U.S. patent covering a bioadhesive technology that would deliver small amounts of N-9 at a consistent rate over a period of twenty-four hours when applied internally. Columbia Labs also discovered that this time-release technique of delivery increased the effectiveness of small doses of N-9 to the degree that the concentration of N-9 needed to kill microorganisms dropped as much as a thousandfold. David Weinberg, who was largely responsible for developing the kit for Columbia Labs, told a London newspaper that "We have found a way of giving a dose that is low enough to avoid sores but high enough to kill infective organisms," generating an effective solution to the previously held concern of N-9 ulceration.[2] Marketed as a commercial contraceptive product to prevent pregnancy under the brand name Advantage 24, the product has been available throughout the United States and Canada for over-the-counter purchase since the early 1990s. Researchers estimated the dependability of the product's protective qualities to be twenty-four hours from the time of application, hence the origin of the brand name.

The development of a promising product that could theoretically be used not only for contraception, but for HIV prophylaxis as well, has renewed the interest and possibility of developing a topical microbicide for rectal use. The bioadhesive nature of Advantage 24, for example, allows the substance to cling to the anal lining (mucosa). Again, however, the public discourse surrounding microbicides for sexual use regularly omits this exciting and noteworthy possibility. In a 1996 press release issued at the Eleventh International Conference on AIDS, U.S. Health and Human Services Secretary Donna Shalala detailed the United States' pledge to triple its monetary commitment to research into topical microbicides. The release stated, "Shalala also called on other developed nations to increase their commitment to microbicide research and asked pharmaceutical manufacturers to make the development of microbicides a priority. 'The development of safe and effective microbicides will give women around the world the power to protect themselves against HIV without fear of abuse or condemnation,' Shalala said."[3] The press release consistently frames microbicides as being "female-controlled" and "used by women," never mentioning the possibility for rectal use or potential benefits to gay men.

As with the female condom, there have been only a few media asides that belie scientists's pondering of the anal application of this technology. For example, in an article trumpeting the United States' commitment to microbicide development, *The Boston Globe* also mentioned, "The same approach, perhaps with different ingredients, might also prevent transmission of HIV and other diseases during anal intercourse between heterosexual or homosexual partners."[4] But some of the obvious anatomical differences between the rectum and vagina continue to pose serious questions about the effectiveness and feasibility of a chemical barrier for safer anal sex. In addition, the sexual landscape of gay male cultures has shifted in such a way that the need for additional forms of protection is more urgent now than ever.

THE NEED FOR RECTAL HARM REDUCTION

In the early 1980s, gay men developed a set of standards for protection from an unknown illness that seemed to be spreading rapidly, claiming lives in the wake of confusion and fear. Even before the virus known as HIV was identified in 1984 and determined to be the cause of subsequent illnesses, a handful of community activists invented the strategy of safer sex to allow sexually active gay men a means by which to reduce their risk of exposure to the suspected pathogen causing "gay cancer." Those standards were incredibly effective in reducing the rates of infection between men, especially in the HIV epicenters of densely populated urban gay communities. Over the following years, however, the imperfections of safer sex became apparent, most notably with respect to condom use for anal sex.

Safer sex was initially conceived and implemented as a stopgap measure. Gay men and others' early faith in medical science to quickly produce an effective treatment, cure, or vaccine eventually proved to be short-sighted. The consistent hope that an end to the mounting toll of death and grief was just around the corner allowed some gay men the tenacity to give up unprotected sex—the only sex they had ever known—and begin to use condoms, abstinence, and mutual monogamy as strategies to avoid HIV. In discussing the time period of 1981 to 1986 as the formational years of risk-reduction strategies we now call safer sex, Cindy Patton has written of the sometimes tenuous relations between scientists' and gay community activists' approaches to combating AIDS:

> Scientists hoped to solve the epidemic through biomedical means, viewing behavioral change as haphazard and impermanent. Activists sought immediate, gay community-controlled behavior change, viewing biomedical intervention as too late for those already infected and too uncertain for those whose infection could be prevented *now*. Scientists hoped biomedical intervention would reduce the harm caused by the virus after infection; activist educators hoped behavioral intervention would prevent transmission in the first place.[5]

As a gradual realization has set in that the stopgap premise would need to become the long-haul norm for gay men to protect themselves, many AIDS educators have realized the need to retool their prevention methodology, as in the case of the absolutist, highly-flawed message of "use a condom every time."

As the basics of AIDS and safer sex education were presumed to be common knowledge among gay men by the late 1980s, new infections in the 1990s have been increasingly characterized both within and outside gay communities as irresponsible, careless, fatalistic, immature, selfish, reckless, and hedonistic. Younger gay men have disproportionately suffered from this judgment, particularly those who had never been sexually active in a time without AIDS and could not claim to have been infected "before they knew better." Many community members and AIDS-prevention specialists attempted (and unfortunately continue) to use a combination of sexual shaming, peer pressure, and fear-based coercion to create a culture of rigid adherence in which a single absence of condom use is met with harsh admonishment rather than honest discussion and caring support.

It should come as no surprise that a cultural phenomenon of conscious and sometimes defiant resistance to safer sex has emerged among some gay men, both HIV negative and positive. But the practice of anal sex without condoms should not be cast purely as a form of backlash against the attempted construction of a specific normative sexuality. Since the early 1990s, social scientists have slowly begun to unpack the multiplicity of motivators and reasons why many gay men continue to engage in unprotected anal intercourse.[6] The complexity of gay male sexuality, infused with a lifetime of homophobic socialization and AIDS-related trauma, defies the popular media's common, sensational portrayal of unsafe sex as a new trend of soundbite-sexy menace and murder.

The unwillingness of policymakers, journalists, AIDS-prevention specialists, and community leaders to acknowledge the valuable meanings of anal sex and body fluid exchange, in all their physical pleasures and cultural significance, has fashioned a popularized rhetoric that is as reductive as it is misguided. Perhaps the most codified illustration of this misunderstanding lies in the public discourse surrounding the practice of barebacking. Most commonly defined, barebacking is the intentional, premeditated, and eroticized act of unprotected anal sex. Reports of barebacking parties and online computer chatrooms dedicated to individuals interested in barebacking have become commonplace. Both HIV-negative and -positive men participate in this activity, as both receptive and insertive partners.

Both gay and mainstream national media (they are becoming increasingly indistinguishable) in the United States have jumped on the barebacking bandwagon, constructing it as the perfect vehicle with which to smear the queers who might decide to forgo condoms. In July 1997, journalist Michelangelo Signorile dedicated his opinion column in *OUT* magazine to the issue, titling it "Bareback and Reckless." Unfortunately Signorile relies predominantly on cyberspace chat room discussions for his research on the topic, then generalizes to an alarmist degree.

For example, mid-way through his column, he reports, "It's impossible to know, however, how widespread the practice of premeditated unprotected sex, for the sheer thrill of it, is among men who engage in anonymous multi-partner sex . . ." but later states with certainty that "it's clearly a growing alarming phenomenon" and refers to barebacking as becoming "more popular" with "a small but growing group of people."[7] He offers no statistical basis for his estimations although he declares them as fact, nor does he address why, if barebacking is becoming so popular, infection rates among most gay male populations have leveled off rather than exploded exponentially. More important, however, is how and where such criticisms take place. Offering a biting critique of Signorile's work, gay activist and scholar Eric Rofes problematizes the scandal approach to bettering gay men's lives. In his book *Dry Bones Breathe: Gay Men Creating Post-AIDS Identities and Cultures,* Rofes responds to Signorile's writing on barebacking by stating, "Rather than address the complexity, Signorile delivers quick sound-bite solutions to vexing social problems. Pointing a finger makes good copy and sells books; it fails to reflect useful processes of self-critique while encouraging the deepening of community divisions."[8]

In addition to *OUT* magazine, *The Advocate* offered a similar take on barebacking months later in February of 1998, although this time the opinion column was not penned by a gay male journalist but rather a heterosexual woman named Kate Shindle, better known as Miss America. Since her crowning in the previous year, Shindle had adopted the platform of AIDS as her form of community service during her pageant reign. Her Viewpoint column, titled "Barebacking? Brainless," attempted to address the possibility that new combination, antiviral therapies might be contributing to a false sense of security and thus increased risk behavior. She asked, "Given the knowledge of what causes the spread of HIV and what we need to do to stop it, how can *we* put ourselves in grave danger and then give it a cute nickname like 'barebacking'? (Italics mine.) Of course the federal government won't fund condom distribution. *We* don't use condoms when *we* have them."[9] (Italics mine.)

At the time of publication, the only published work suggesting that protease inhibitor success could be contributing to unsafe behavior were studies conducted with gay men. The survey was conducted by the University of California San Francisco's Center for AIDS Prevention Studies and included only fifty-four men from one urban area. The results were published as a letter to the editor of the *New England Journal of Medicine*, not as a peer-reviewed study, and noted, "The interviews confirmed that for most participants, information about the 'new treatments' did not reduce their level of concern about infection or their perception of the risk of infection."[10] In addition, there has been no media or scientific reporting of heterosexual subcultures adopting the term barebacking in reference to premeditated, eroticized, unprotected sex.

One is left asking, just who is the "we" that Kate Shindle repeatedly addresses? And on what evidence does she base her declaration that "The translation is clear: We're having unsafe sex now that there's a slim chance that we're closer to the end of this epidemic."[11] Traditionally idolized by many gay men, Miss America has gone from campy diva to sexual disciplinarian. Aside from Shindle's misinformed assumptions, her lack of an intricate understanding of gay male cultures and chastising of gay male sexuality (in a gay publication, no less) belies a tension of broader social relations. As epitomized in the above examples, the queer barebacker has become the latest posterchild of infectious demonization; he is scapegoated and held responsible for everything from loss of government AIDS-prevention dollars to the supposed decay of urban gay male culture. As the embodiment of all AIDS-prevention frustrations, he defies not only state regulation of sexuality, but the very constitution of gay men as Architects of Safer Sex and AIDS-Caregiving Angels.[12]

But even in the gay media, there is a great reluctance to publicly acknowledge and discuss the integral meanings of anal sex that are so fundamental to many gay men's identities and lives. The treatment of anal sex as something inherently disposable, easily replace-able, and casually elective have missed the mark of effective HIV-risk reduction by such a distance that many AIDS-prevention specialists continue to ask, "If they're not under the influence of a chemical substance, depressed, or stupid, why would gay men have unprotected anal sex in this day and age?" Regardless of the outrage expressed by media and community leaders, and despite any at-tempts to intervene with state authority, some gay men will continue to have unprotected anal sex for a variety and complexity of rea-sons. In the tradition of safer sex and needle-exchange programs, there exists a clear and urgent need for barebacking risk-reduction strategies. This has become a dangerous proposition, and even the public discussions of microbicides for vaginal use are careful to remind readers that such a chemical barrier would not be intended to serve as the only method of protection:

> The goal is not to find a substitute for condom use, said Dr. Christopher Elias of The Population Council, an international nonprofit agency devoted to reproductive health research. "Negotiating condom use, however, is not always feasible," he said. "Women often have too little power within their sexual relationships to insist on condom use, and they often have too little power outside of these relationships to abandon partners that put them at risk."[13]

This excerpt from a *Boston Globe* article typifies the commonplace, qualitative distinction made between sexual partners in socioeco-nomic situations who are, in a variety of ways, forced and coerced to engage in unprotected sex versus those sexual partners who make conscious choices to engage in such activity without fear of abuse or abandonment by their partner.

In an interesting departure from the norm of state conservatism, in 1992 the New York State Health Department created a brochure titled "For Women Only." The brochure targeted women who faced difficulty in convincing their male partners to use condoms for vaginal sex, and gave suggestions for nonlatex condom alternatives, arranged along a spectrum of safety. At the riskiest end of the spectrum, the brochure suggests the use of a spermicidal product alone as "better than nothing." As the cleverly titled article in *Vil-*

lage Voice, "Iffy Lube," pointed out, "This was an unusual recommendation from a public agency. Most have taken their lead from the Centers for Disease Control, which does not endorse the use of N-9 without condoms for HIV prevention. Still, the DOH [Department of Health] recommendations may reflect the fact that New York City has the highest concentration of AIDS cases [in the state of New York]."[14] In contrast, however, the Department of Health refused to make any recommendation about the rectal use of N-9, even in similar situations where men may have difficulty convincing their male partners to use condoms for anal sex. The panel that decided not to take action on rectal recommendations cited a lack of research as a justification for inaction, but as Richard Elovich, Director of HIV Prevention at Gay Men's Health Crisis, told the *Village Voice,* "That's a catch-22 . . . If a panel of public health experts doesn't identify this as an issue, how is it going to get researched?"[15]

Rather than waiting for sanctioned government approval to make recommendations about the use of microbicides and other noncondom tactics for minimizing risk of infection, some community groups have decided to take matters into their own hands. The suggestion of a movement to minimize the harm associated with willful barebacking has already generated the classic wave of shock and outcry from those who believe that promotion of risk reduction strategies will only serve to legitimize and condone such behavior. In 1998, the People with AIDS Coalition in Ft. Lauderdale came under attack for their dissemination of these strategies in their monthly newsletter.[16] For the most part, their suggested practices for risk reduction consisted of behavioral strategies divorced from technological aid, including early withdrawal before ejaculation, counseling, proper lubrication to reduce tearing, and more. Again, gay communities run the risk of recreating an artificial separation of biomedical, cultural, and behavioral approaches to this work that Cindy Patton and others have mapped and critiqued in a historical context. How might we create, appropriate, or even imagine certain technologies as means of risk reduction for those gay men who choose, for a multitude of reasons, to engage in anal sex without condoms?

Rather than abiding by the divisiveness of behavioral versus biomedical approaches to risk reduction, why not seek the development of synergistic collaborations between the two? In a 1997 opinion editorial published in the San Francisco gay newspaper *Bay Area Reporter*, Clark Taylor makes such a call:

> It is astounding to me that as good as we are at getting drugs tested, we have done nothing to get scientists to create rectal chemical barriers to STDs. This is in stark contrast to the work being done on vaginal microbicides! Women have been extremely effective in getting new products researched and tested. But we have been almost completely silent about our needs. . . . We must insist that research on rectal microbicides begin immediately and with enough funding to see that it proceeds quickly.[17]

Taylor is a senior researcher at the Institute for Advanced Study of Sexuality and serves as a consultant who is frequently contracted to conduct microbicide research for universities, corporations, and government organizations.

In an attempt to gain a better sense of the issues related to microbicides that might not be reflected in published literature and other available textual data, I conducted interviews with Taylor and another scientist, Connie Celum, to further discern some of the politics and prospects of rectal microbicides for gay men. Celum is part of an organization called the HIV Network of Vaccine Efficacy Trials (HIVNET). Established in 1993 by the National Institute of Allergy and Infectious Disease (NIAID), HIVNET's purpose is to lay the groundwork and coordinate efficacy trials of HIV-prevention strategies that are primarily clinical and biomedical in nature. In addition to vaccine research, HIVNET is responsible for evaluating the effectiveness of other interventions aimed at preventing the spread of HIV, including vaginal and anal microbicides. Celum works with HIVNET in addition to holding a faculty position at the University of Washington in Seattle. She was also the principle investigator of a Phase I clinical trial involving the use of a N-9 (Advantage 24) for anal use in men, whereas Taylor has recently been working on a different kind of microbicide, the effectiveness of which hinges upon an acid-buffering agent.

The content and comparison of my interviews with these two scientists offer some interesting insights with respect to some of the basic research approaches and politicized meanings attached to rectal microbicides and anal sexual health. In the interview quotes throughout the rest of this chapter, "MS" indicates my comments and questions, "CC" denotes Connie Celum, and "CT" are the statements of Clark Taylor.

RECTAL MICROBICIDE RESEARCH AND DEVELOPMENT

Clark Taylor agreed to meet with me during my visit to San Francisco in early 1998, and I interviewed him one afternoon at a small restaurant in the Castro neighborhood. I began by asking Taylor to explain his current work and how he came to be interested in microbicides, particularly those for rectal use.

> **CT:** My research is through my capacity as a senior research at the IASHS and also as an independent contractor. I was contracted by the San Francisco AIDS Foundation in 1982 to research the information on how to use condoms and to create a document that could be made into some kind of pamphlet for information use. In the process, our Institute had done some preliminary research on Trimensa's ForePlay, with 1 percent N-9 in it and rectal gonorrhea. That research was never finished, but the Institute was probably the first group that introduced me to the idea of chemical prophylaxis or topical microbicides. . . . Bruce Voller, of the Mariposa Foundation, was at that time saying we should take a look at spermicides as a viable adjunct or layer of risk reduction for rectal intercourse. It's true [the rectum] is a tube, and an open-ended tube, but if you put in enough, it will coat it.

Taylor pursued these ideas over time and sought out networking opportunities with scientists, activists, and policymakers who shared similar interests and recognized the potential of chemical prophylaxis against sexually transmitted infections.

CT: When I would go to the International AIDS conferences, I would look for possible products and people interested in the area [of microbicides] and I began to discover papers that were very interesting. I quickly zeroed in on a number of possibilities and a number of issues that turned out to be quite right. I also had the good luck to find out about a meeting being held in Santo Domingo in 1992 by the Population Council, the National Institutes of Science, and various other world organizations on topical microbicides and the prevention of STDs. I went there, and that was when it really got exciting. There's a big split in AIDS research between the people doing topical microbicide work and the people doing drug research and treatment. In fact, I found there was very little communication between both groups and very little understanding of one another's work.

The "big split" to which Taylor refers is somewhat classic in health sciences. In this case, the split is between topical microbicides and other pharmaceutical work, but more broadly it mirrors the problematic divide between prevention and treatment. Celum echoed Taylor's observation and discussed the prioritization of treatment over prevention in AIDS research.

MS: Do you have any speculation or thoughts on AIDS activism and why it's been so effective in pushing for new and better HIV treatments, but not for the development of new safer sex technologies?

CC: My personal perspective is that, in general, prevention is sort of the underrecognized stepchild. Treatment has a more politicized group. It's easier to find who has an investment in trying to find treatments, whereas when you're talking about prevention, there isn't as strong an interest or definable community that's going to make a cry for HIV vaccines, microbicides, or a number of other prevention strategies. I think this is clearly true in the area of HIV vaccines as well. There's been an effort to develop advocacy for development and testing of HIV vaccines, but it's still small and not nearly as vocal as the advocates for treatment initiatives.

Celum also articulated the progress of her research and offered her opinions on the future of such biomedical pursuits by outlining some of the more basic concepts and issues that will frame this work for years to come:

MS: Why is the research and development of rectal microbicides so important to current HIV prevention?

CC: Well, first of all, maybe as a backup we should ask why microbicides are important in general, because the issues for vaginal and rectal microbicides are very similar. Basically, the idea behind microbicides is to try to find compounds, biochemical products that have either an antiseptic effect, in other words sterilize the environment of the vagina or rectum and ideally would work against HIV and then some of the other STD pathogens like gonorrhea, chlamydia, herpes, in particular. The idea is that since condoms aren't always used, and when they are used they're not always used properly, or sometimes they break or slip, so instead of a mechanical barrier, this is a chemical barrier to try to protect primarily the receptive partner against infection with these compounds. The whole area of microbicide development is one that's gotten a lot of press over the last couple of years. Frankly, it's a very early kind of science and I think we're learning as we do these kind of clinical trials in humans that there is a whole host of issues that still need to be worked out in terms of what are that biologic properties of the active ingredient that you want, how do you deliver it. If you found an effective product, you'd also have to really deal with acceptability to make sure that it was something that has the right kind of lubricating properties and something that is acceptable to both the receptive and insertive partner. So there are a whole host of those issues too, and I think that we're learning as we do the study that we're at the very early end of the development process in terms of understanding what are the right issues, and how do you address them, and product development and clinical trials.

GENDERED AND ANATOMICAL COMPARISONS

As I have discussed my research on this topic with a variety of individuals, the most common comment I have encountered is the comparison of open-ended and closed-ended body cavities. There is a great deal of skepticism as to whether or not an effective vaginal microbicide could be adapted for anal use in a way that would provide thorough coverage of the rectal mucosa. Author and AIDS activist Rob Gorna explains:

> One question, which is rarely asked, is whether microbicides would work only in the vagina, or also in the anus? Most data on microbicides discusses their use for vaginal intercourse. This is principally because the vagina has the form of a "pouch"—which can be fully line by a product and contain it—whereas the anus is "open-ended," so that a product may not be contained within the rectum and could leak up into the intestines. Microbicide research also appears to concentrate on the vagina because of the general prurience and neglect of the anus as a sexual organ.[18]

In a poster presentation made at the 12th World AIDS Conference in Geneva, Switzerland in 1998, Clark Taylor posed a series of additional questions out of concern for the suitability of a vaginal product to be adopted for rectal use. These included: Is defecation necessary before inserting the substance? Should it be "voided" after sex (if even possible)? How might rectal absorption effect efficacy?[19]

In the meeting minutes of HIVNET's microbicide committee, the same issues have repeatedly been mulled, generating another set of perspectives:

> In discussing the concept of advancing only promising vaginal products in rectal studies, it was suggested that some of the requirements for vaginal use of these products, e.g., spermicidal activity, are not relevant to rectal use, and that products that may not be promising for vaginal use may be suitable for rectal use. Provided there is strong support by a manufacturer, these should remain under consideration."[20]

Based on some of these statements in HIVNET documents, I posed a more pointed question to Celum regarding this ongoing concern.

MS: The vagina, in some ways, seems better suited for a more full protective coating by a microbicide due to its enclosed structure, whereas the rectum is more open-ended. Because of that open-endedness, how or would a rectal microbicide fully protect the rectum?

CC: We don't know. No one really knows. As I've learned more, I think it's amazing that some of these vaginal products have been out there—contraceptive foams and jellies. The distribution properties really haven't been worked out that well. It's amazing they didn't have to go through a lot of rigorous testing. So they're out there, but as we look at various thing like the N-9 film, creams, and suppositories, there are a lot of questions that we don't have answers for even with vaginal products, let alone rectal. I think the issues are going to be different and the challenges will be somewhat different to find a product that does coat a thick enough area of the mucosa to offer protection, but we don't know exactly what the target amount of protection should be, because we don't know how high up semen really can go, and where infection occurs when it does happen. So there are certain unknowns that we'll probably always be faced with, but I think the challenge with rectal microbicides will be getting enough product that coats well, but is not too big of a volume in terms of just the discomfort of fullness that some men will experience.

MS: What are perhaps some of the possible advantages and disadvantages of developing a microbicide that is specific to the rectum and not for vaginal use as well?

CC: I don't think there will be microbicides likely developed just for rectal use, because I think the delivery systems may be different, although I think these are commercial companies that are only going to probably put their investment and resources into something which can be used by a wider population. I think the lube companies don't have the scientific structure to really get into microbicide development in any kind of serious way. The people who have been involved with N-9 and some of the other products are either commercial entities—their background is focused on vaginal products—or agencies that are looking at products for both contraceptive and disease protection roles, like Population Council. So I think it's unlikely that you're going to see a lot of resources put into just looking for products for rectal use.

The economic market for microbicides, above all else, has consistently surfaced as the primary dictator of prospective development and viability. The commercial nature of this gamble involves pumping research dollars into a product that would eventually return not only the development investment, but a longterm and worthwhile profit to the corporations seeking to capitalize on such a product. The competition between entities who seek to patent a successful product has lead to a slight diversification in the kinds of substances being investigated for internal use, but the market limits of this developmental breadth have yet to be tested.

An article in a 1997 issue of the trade publication *Drug Store News* reported:

> Unfortunately, while all indications suggest that the market is ripe for sharp increases in the sale of over-the-counter contraceptive products, particularly condoms, the actual sales figures tell a different story. The category is relatively flat and has been for quite some time. . . . By rethinking merchandising schemes, chain drug stands to increase its contraceptive sales as the suppliers work to draw new users to the category.[21]

Drawing new users to the category does not necessarily mean the adaptation or creation of new safer sex technologies, however; nor does it entail courting a sizeable gay market.

Lake Consumer Products Inc., the marketer and distributor of Advantage 24, launched a national ad campaign for their microbicide, intended to reach "some 70 million women via print, and, starting in the fall [of 1997] cable television commercials will be reaching over 31 million women via Lifetime, E!, Comedy Central,

VH1, and other channels skewed toward females."[22] Rather than using gender-neutral programming that could appeal to a broader range of sexualities and relationships, the decidedly female-specific targeting excludes gay men from this market in a number of ways, similar to the marketing used by the Female Health Company's campaign for the Reality Female Condom.

In November 1997, Reuters newswire service released a story touting the achievement of a team of Canadian researchers who had formulated a liquid condom that could be applied to the body, hardening and molding to the skin's surface. One news piece explained that:

> Developed over seven years by Laval University's Infectious Diseases Research Center, the new "condom" is in fact a nontoxic polymer-based liquid that solidifies into a gel at body temperature. A woman or male homosexual partner would apply the liquid to genital or anal parts before a sexual encounter. Laval said tests showed that the gel formed a water-proof film that dramatically reduced transmission of the AIDS virus and could also block the virus responsible for genital herpes.[23]

This is an example of a more physical than chemical kind of barrier, but represents one more possibility in scientific efforts to create condom alternatives. As promising as these ongoing discoveries continue to be, the gap remains large between laboratory prototypes and commercial products with unrestricted consumer access. Taylor told me that:

> **CT:** I've discussed with various companies strategies given that there is such a tremendous difficulty in any Western country developing and marketing and selling a rectal product other than for piles and things like that. No one wants to touch it. It's not viable enough, and these companies openly say so.

TYPES OF MICROBICIDES

There are many different types of potential microbicides for the prevention of sexually transmitted infections. I have chosen a few of those currently under study that look to be at least somewhat promising, based on interviews and available documents. Briefly outlined below, they represent how radically different substances might be employed to accomplish similar chemical tasks of prophylaxis.

Acid-Buffering

An acid-buffering microbicide would essentially alter the pH level of the tissue to be protected. This could be especially useful against HIV, which does not survive as long when pH levels are lowered. Daily vaginal suppositories, designed to lower pH by raising levels of natural vaginal microflora that would be hostile to pathogens, are currently under development. BufferGel, the brand name of an acid-buffering microbicide, was cleared by the Food and Drug Administration (FDA) in 1996 for Phase I clinical trials and was the first AIDS-prevention technology to be chosen by HIVNET for clinical trials. At the time of my interview with him, Clark Taylor was working with a Johns Hopkins University's research project which formed a company called ReProtect, investigating microbicides that contained acid-buffering agents. He further explained to me:

> **CT:** Semen and blood are extremely good neutralizing buffers that bring the acidity of the vagina up to [a pH level of] seven, and keep it there for many hours. That's how conception takes place. One of the several ways that the buffering gel works is that it maintains a low level of acid pH in the presence of semen and blood and other kinds of neutralizing agents. Acidity kills most every pathogen. The problem has been finding something that has the certain kinds of characteristics including, and most important, the ability to buffer. Other kinds of acidic agents—they will acidify for a while but then they fail.

Nonoxynol-9 (N-9)

As discussed earlier in this chapter, perhaps the most promising commercial product utilizing N-9 seems to be Advantage 24. In fact, the only products on the market that were ready for efficacy trials in 1997 were those that contained N-9. Celum's Phase I study of Advantage 24, conducted in Seattle with gay men practicing anal intercourse, is significant because it may, for the first time, yield reliable data on rectal safety of N-9 exposure in humans. This information holds additional importance because many sexual lubricants sold over the counter and marketed to gay men also contain the same compound that is used to form its adhesive base. But the mixture of Advantage 24 with condoms, however, raises some troubling complications, as noted by Taylor:

> **CT:** Advantage 24 is identical to Replens, the vaginal moisturizer. Both products have mineral oil in them. Columbia [corporation] contracted out to test the burst strength of condoms used with Advantage 24, but they stacked the deck, meaning they applied it to condoms for five minutes, with no friction or heat, then submitted them to the burst test, found they reduced the condom effectiveness by 30 percent as compared to the controls, but the [condom] strength was still above the bare government standards.

The effectiveness of delivering any microbicide will remain dependent on the other ingredients of the product and how they might interact when used with existing safer sex technologies. The success or failure of N-9 remains hanging within the indelicate balance between toxicity and antiviral impact.

Others

In addition to the previous two, an assortment of other substances have attracted researchers' attention due to the possibility of their microbicidal properties. Taylor was especially well-versed in the vast array of these contemporary inquiries. Among them are carragean and a compound known as C31G.

> **CT:** Carragean is used primarily in foods as a thickener. May make it possible to have a microbicide that does not prevent pregnancy very well, but does entrap and neutralize HIV. It may or may not work for other STDs. It appears to work with

hepatitis and some viruses. . . . C31G is two surfactants which, when mixed together, have antibiotic properties. It's used in mouthwash available through dentists, not available to the general public, for stopping pyorrhea. N-9 sterilizes an area, but doesn't permit healing. C31G not only sterilizes but also seems to promote healing.

No doubt there will be future research into the existing substances that demonstrate promising utility in addition to the new compounds that are engineered specifically for such purposes at hand.

PROSPECTIVE POLITICS

As with the politics embedded in other issues of protective technologies for anal sex described in this book, microbicides are not exempt from being mired in larger struggles of power and control. In 1996, a San Francisco activist sent out a press release concerning the need for rectal microbicides to a number of media, and one of them—*The Washington Times*—responded. The activist chose to garner attention by framing microbicide research as a dire necessity for gay male sexual health. As is typical with such media coverage, however, a more personified controversy is needed to make the material newsworthy, so *Washington Times* reporter Joyce Price initiated contact with a few spokespersons for conservative organizations, presented them with information about rectal microbicide clinical trials underway in Seattle, and solicited their opinion. With little substantive knowledge of the issue at hand, at least two of them offered their predictable opinion on the matter:

> "We are facilitating, at taxpayer expense, an illegal and immoral activity that's abhorrent to most Americans. . . . If we make homosexual sex safer, all we're going to do is promote promiscuity, which will lead to more STDs," said Bob Maginnis, senior policy analyst for the Family Research Council.
> The Rev. Lou Sheldon, chairman of the Traditional Values Coalition, had this reaction to the Phase I Rectal Microbicide Study: "Perversion is perversion any way you try to rewrite it. The funding of this kind of study is inappropriate and really

goes against the beliefs and values of a significant majority of Americans."[24]

While Maginnis fell back on the tired equation of "homosexuality equals promiscuity equals disease," Sheldon attempted to invoke the will of the imagined majority. Perhaps most interesting is the absence of any expressed commitment to action, as neither Maginnis nor Sheldon threatened to boycott, lobby, protest, or otherwise organize around this issue. A few well-placed sound bites sufficed to generate the appearance of opposition and lend personality to the orchestrated controversy.

During my interview with Celum, I could not resist a solicitation of her opinion on the polemical, albeit brief, journalism surrounding the study.

> **MS:** I came across last year's *Washington Times* article in my literature search. I was curious: how did the right-wing organizations even find out about the study? And secondly, has there been any substantive impact from the media publicity and the backlash surrounding that?

> **CC:** From what I understand, there is an activist who has been trying to get more attention and funding for the whole area of rectal microbicides over the last couple of years, and would show up at national meetings and say, "The NIH should be funding more rectal microbicide studies" and learned of our study, which was NIH-funded. I think he wanted to make a point of it to encourage healthy debate that this is a reasonable area to study and get more funding allocated for this. In the process, apparently he called a number of newspapers and the only one that bit the story was *The Washington Times*. So we tried to do our best at explaining the rationale and of course they selectively reported what they wanted to and interviewed the other groups. But there really was very little backlash. We were all poised for this to lead to Congressional hew and cry. The timing worked out so that it made a little blip, and we all sort of waited nervously, and nothing came of it, so we finished the study. Maybe if it was publicized more widely at a different time at a Congressional cycle, it might have made a

different impact. . . . The reporter asked questions like, "Are
you paying men to have sex?"

I think the conservative groups said no, they didn't like it,
when they were interviewed, but they certainly didn't do anything that I'm aware of to try to block it. There's one state
legislator in Washington who somehow heard about it and
wrote a fairly mild letter, in my opinion, to the dean of the
School of Medicine here to say, "Is this our state tax payer
dollar going toward this?" and that was an easy thing to answer.

In this case, the federal nature of the funding source spared the
study from an intensity of scrutinization at the state and local political levels. Luckily, the prospect of increased federal funding for this
kind of work looks somewhat promising. For example, in July
1997, the Centers for Disease Control and Prevention publicized the
availability of funding for epidemiological and behavioral research
studies of HIV and AIDS. Their announcement stated,

The purpose of these awards is to help support researchers in
the conduct of HIV-related epidemiologic and behavioral research studies that foster prevention of HIV infection and HIV
related disease. These include . . . studies to examine behavioral and biomedical factors related to the acceptability of new
products to prevent sexual transmission of HIV infection such
as vaginal and rectal microbicides.

Under a section delineating specific research issues, men who have
sex with men are a focus population from which to collect survey
data on the "extent to which prevention methods being tested (e.g.,
products that could be used as rectal microbicide) are desirable, and
the conditions under which these methods would be chosen."[25]
While this sort of funding may become more readily available in
the future, the stigma attached to such work may discourage experts
from tapping it as a resource. As the Seattle study demonstrated,
even the basic inquiry about an individual and relatively small-scale
study was enough to make the principle investigators nervous, hoping the attention would subside rather than generate inflammatory
and public debate. But it's not just conservative right-wing organi-

zations or popular sentiment that are problematic obstacles in conducting this research or securing funding in support of future work in the area. Later in our interview, Celum discussed the scarcity of scientists who are willing to tackle studies that are central to issues of sexuality and sexual behavior, especially deviant behavior such as anal sex and homosexuality. In her opinion, "Most of the researchers in this field aren't just homophobic, they are erotophobic." With extremely rare exceptions, sexuality as a field of scientific inquiry does not hold promise for those researchers and academics who seek to establish mainstream legitimacy, high levels of grant funding, or the prominence of prestigeous awards.

Encouraging results from studies on rectal microbicides will likely be painstakingly incremental. As the only one of its kind to date, the stated objective of HIVNET's N-9 study in Seattle was "to assess safety, acceptability, and effect of nonoxynol-9 (N-9) on rectal viral STDs when used as a topical rectal microbicide." As of April 1997, thirty-four of the thirty-five couples who initially enrolled had completed the study. There was minimal inflammation as the result of product use, and the most frequent complaint was that of rectal fullness reported by the receptive partners, meaning the experience of a nongaseous bloating sensation.[26]

> **MS:** Obviously this was a Phase I study. Could you define for me what a Phase II and Phase III study would look like if they occur in the future?
>
> **CC:** Well, Phase II would be looking at safety and acceptability issues in a higher-risk population, the kind of target population you would enroll in a Phase III efficacy study. Probably you would not be enrolling couples, but just enrolling individuals who are likely going to use a rectal microbicide and would be counseled in Phases II and III to also use condoms. But you would know that, as a number of studies have documented, people don't always use condoms all the time, so we would be encouraging them to use this at least as a backup when they don't use condoms. You would probably also not screen out men who had gonorrhea and chlamydia, HIV-negative men who had herpes. So, we really were looking at very low risk, basically monogamous couples in the Phase I study,

and we would not have that stringent eligibility criteria in Phases II or III.

MS: Is there a Phase II study planned for the near future?

CC: No, not at this point. I think the whole strategy of when you do rectal studies versus vaginal studies based on the incredible number of resources to do any kind of human clinical trials, I think what's likely going to happen will be to do Phases I and II studies of vaginal products and perhaps after the Phase II, then do Phases I and II rectally. I think these are going to be targeted for both vaginal and rectal use. There's much more experience doing vaginal studies. It's a little bit easier to know where the product is, and know that it hasn't gone further into the rectum, and so on. I think the first safety and acceptability questions will be asked in terms of vaginal use and then, with promising products, go on to rectal use. I think what we'll find with microbicides will be similar to vaccines—that some products will fall off because they have too high of a toxicity to the epithelium or the volume is so high that the acceptability is not great, so it makes sense to do step-wise approaches and use what limited resources there are for microbicides judiciously, to not plan that everything is going to go into an efficacy trial, because certainly there just aren't enough cohorts or resources to really be able to do efficacy trials, which are likely going to be three or four thousand person studies. I mean, they're huge studies.

In one survey conducted with Brazilian gay men, "Among 61 subjects reporting receptive anal intercourse, twenty-eight (46 percent) expressed a willingness to participate in studies of a rectal microbicide containing nonoxynol-9."[27] If this serves as any indication of larger scale research attempts, funding will likely remain the chief obstacle to efficacy trials rather than a lack of voluntary trial participants.

LEFT TO OUR OWN DEVICES

So where does all of this confusion, inaction, reluctance, and unexplored possibility leave gay men? Clark Taylor believes the reality of the near future will somewhat mirror that of the female condom, saying that, "There is only one FDA route right now to get a product on the market, and that is to have a spermicide for vaginal use that also has the ability to stop STDs." Similar to Celum's expectation of the only possible advancement, gay men will likely be left to fend for themselves, crossing the gender lines of drugstore marketing to appropriate yet another vaginal product for rectal use. In fact, Taylor says he knows several gay men who are already doing just that. He told me of men who are buying and using Advantage 24 over-the-counter for rectal use, both in lieu of and in addition to condoms.

Why is it that gay men can conceptualize this form of appropriation and take the risks involved with the adaptation of these products, but not organize around this problematic void to improve safer sex technologies and access to them? Taylor speculates:

> **CT:** Part of the reason we don't mobilize around this issue is that we haven't really conceived of it. There's a strong naiveté that if something is developed for the vagina it will work for the mouth and rectum. Obviously that's not true. There are many different issues. The flora and fauna are different; the cells are much more delicate in the rectum; the receptor cells are very different.

Despite some misunderstanding surrounding the science of topical microbicides, a few organizations have formed to lobby federal agencies and legislators for the advancement of this research, most notably a group calling themselves Microbicides As an Alternative Solution (MAS), based out of the Center for Family and Community Health at University of California, Berkeley. Their stated mission reads:

> Each sexual partner should have the ability to protect him/herself from HIV and STDs. Our organization advocates for the development of accessible and affordable methods (i.e., microbicides) for HIV and STD prevention *for people who do not currently have a method they can control.* We educate the public, policy-makers and research institutions about the urgent need for innovative prevention methods.[27] (Italics mine)

Once again, the need for microbicides is cast in a dire light of absent alternatives and lack of control over one's own sexual experience. It may make for a compelling letter to one's congressman, but creates an argument that is restrictive in its reasoning for access to improved sexual technologies. Both men and women who have access to condoms and engage in consensual, noncoercive sexual activity are presumed not to need these products.

Although rectal microbicide development is included in the group's broader agenda, it is not a priority, and the alliance is not a gay organization per se. The need for specific advocacy and lobbying around anal pleasure and health in this area is clear, although no major gay health organization or activist group has prioritized this need as part of their main agenda. As Clark Taylor noted at the close of my interview with him, "The most astonishing and reprehensible thing—and I don't know any way to address it—is why, when we as a gay community have so much to gain with this kind of development and so much to lose without it, we raise not a voice to either advocate it or influence policy or anything."

SECTION III:
THE SMEAR FOR MICROSCOPIC
EXAMINATION

A Recipe for Rectal Tarts
(or, Just Add Feces and Stir)

First concocted in the experimental kitchens of Paul Cameron's Family Research Institute, this recipe is perfect for today's busy and healthy lifestyle. It's a steamy dish sure to become a chosen family favorite!

His name is Chef Paul Cameron,
culinary wiz of our day.
Promiscuity and gay men
make his moral dish quite gourmet.

He cooks up hazards of queerness,
finding danger in tarts of fruit—
recipes for peril from the
Family Research Institute.

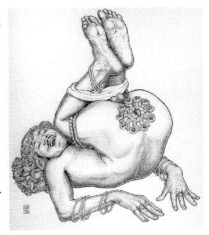

"The rectum is a mixing bowl"*
for a rich medley of disease—
chosen-family favorites,
made for multiple guests with ease.

Rectal tarts are guilty pleasures
much more decadent than Sodom.
Their heat is sure to be scorching,
so take care to grease the bottom.

Illustration by Kira Od.

And please don't forget the rimming,
or the bowl just won't be the same.
Clean-as-you-go is the rule here,
and hygiene the name of the game.

Next, blend together a mishmash
of semen, lube, and saliva.
This confection of infection
is much sweeter than Godiva.

Allow to rise until the stick
which is inserted comes out clean.
Avoid overbrowning the top;
this results in Tarts a Latrine.

Sprinkle the top with parasites.
(Amoebas will do in a pinch.)
With incubation in minutes,
these savory snacks are a cinch!

Easily shared with others and
a course best prepared in the home,
such pathogens of the colon
are also called "Gay Bowel Syndrome."*

Ideal for any occasion,
unequalled by riced crispy treats,
they're perfect for bath house bake sales
and "biological swap meets."*

---

*These statements and phrases are quoted directly from the pamphlet "Medical Consequences of What Homosexuals Do," written by (not a real) "Dr." Paul Cameron and published by the right-wing homophobe scapegoating organization, The Family Research Institute, 1993.

Chapter 4

Queering the Smear:
A Detective Named Pap

Leafing through the pages of *The Advocate* one afternoon in February of 1995, the words "male Pap smear" leapt out at me from a health column buried inside. The short article appeared in the magazine's front section, dedicated to new and noteworthy tidbits, often of a somewhat sensational nature. Having studied feminist theory of women's health and engaged in conversation with women friends about the procedure, the thought of a male-specific or even gender-neutral version of this gynecological mainstay bore a significance to me that surpassed the realm of medical peculiarity. The article briefly explained, "Some experts now suggest that men with a history of anal receptive intercourse or anal warts should be screened on a regular basis for anal cancer or precancerous lesions."[1] From a first and not-so-careful reading, I supposed the article was suggesting that receptive anal intercourse in some way caused anal cancer and therefore anal Pap smears had become a necessary form of preventive maintenance for gay men's early detection of the disease.

Out of curiosity, I conducted a literature review on anal Pap smears at Ohio State University health sciences library and tracked down a sparse handful of citations. Most of the published research seemed to be highly preliminary in tone, representing an exploratory body of work that introduced seemingly significant results. As I learned more about the topic, I slowly began to evaluate my own risk for anal cancer, as I am someone who has practiced receptive anal intercourse. Eventually, I decided to seek a screening for the condition.

A few months later, in April 1995, I sat in my doctor's office prepared with a collection of medical journal articles that detailed and rationalized anal Pap smears for gay men. I explained to him that a screening for anal cancer seemed worthwhile given my sexual history and requested the test. Although surprised, he was intrigued and open to the idea. Similar to Pap smears for women that detect the possibility of cervical cancer, my procedure was relatively painless, easy, and inexpensive. As *The Advocate* article described, "It consists of inserting a moistened swab at least five centimeters into the anus. The patient is asked to bear down, and the swab is rotated as it is removed."[2] The cells collected with the swab are then quickly preserved on a glass slide for later microscopic analysis, better known as the smear.

The protocol of my particular health care provider, Ohio State University's Student Health Services, required funneling all Pap smears through their Women's Clinic for shipment to an outside laboratory. This gender-specific administrative course struck me as a bit odd, never having imagined a reliance upon gynecological practice for my own wellness, especially my sexual health. (I later learned that the staff of the Women's Clinic were also a bit surprised to receive a male sample for processing.) My physician sent me on my way after the smear was secured, and I proceeded to the clinic's check-out desk with my paperwork for billing and a follow-up appointment. The woman working at the desk entered my data into the computer system, only to be met with an error code that prevented her from processing the completion of my visit. After several unsuccessful attempts to correct the error, she consulted with another staff person. That person was similarly puzzled, and after a great deal of frustration, they summoned the clinic's computer support person. By this time, I was as annoyed as they were, so they told me I could leave, assuring me they would solve the problem later rather than asking me to wait.

When I returned in two weeks for the results of my smear, the same staff person told me that after consulting the manuals that accompany the clinic's computer software, they had found the culprit. It seems the software came embedded with a series of error-checkers, among them a routine cross-check between the patient's profile and the lab tests billed to the patient. If some discord was detected between the patient's gender and a gender-specific medical procedure, the system would flag the entry as incorrect and impede the billing process until corrected. In order to bypass the software, she told me she had resorted to editing my online patient profile, changing my sex to "female," processing my office visit, then changing my profile again back to "male" after the transaction.

While reviewing the results of my Pap smear with me, my physician told me how the lab technician who analyzed the smear had called him more than once. The technician had no real substantive questions about the smear itself, but seemed to be rather disturbed at the thought of conducting an anal Pap smear, and had requested some form of vague reassurance about the procedure. The results of my smear indicated mild dysplasia—slightly abnormal cells that were nothing serious, but something to be monitored over time in case they changed into malignant lesions.

Aside from direct interactions with my physician, my smear troubled and complicated existing systems of medical care at almost every level. I began to wonder why a medical technology that had historically been applied to female bodies should draw such attention when used with gay men. Perhaps naively, the consequences of queering the smear took me by surprise and signified, once again, the tenuous relationship between gendered technologies and sexually deviant bodies. What began as a simple precancer screening turned out to be a prime example of the difficulties gay men continue to face as they advocate for their own specific health care needs within unaccomodating or unprepared frameworks of preventive medicine. In the case of anal cancer, access to screening, assessment, and treatment have become increasingly significant to gay men for a number of reasons.

The prevalence of anorectal cancer appears to be rising in many gay male populations, particularly those with a history of infection with human papillomavirus (HPV) of the anus.[3] HPV infection is sometimes expressed as genital or anal warts that take the shape of a cauliflower-like skin formation (also known as *condyloma acuminata*). In the last fifteen years, the nature of the association between HPV and anal cancer has attracted increasing attention from medical scientists who specialize in the fields of cancer treatment, HIV infection, and to a lesser extent, proctology and gynecology. Many researchers have been reluctant to state that HPV directly causes anal cancer, but agree that HPV plays a strong role in the development of abnormal tissue cells that sometimes develop into cancer.

CARCINOGENIC HOMOSEXUALITY

As in other cases of medical investigation into gay male health problems, a handful of researchers have gone so far as to suggest that homosexuality itself may be a causative agent in the development of bodily disease. Take, for example, two studies conducted by Janet R. Daling of the Fred Hutchinson Cancer Research Center in Seattle, Washington. The first study's findings, "Correlates of Homosexual Behavior and the Incidence of Anal Cancer" were published in a 1982 *Journal of the American Medical Association.* Daling and her colleagues stated, "This study was conducted to explore the possibility that the occurrence of some malignant diseases might be related to male homosexual behavior."[4] The specific "male homosexual behavior" Daling refers to is none other than receptive, unprotected anal intercourse. In the study, it became progressively equated with male homosexuality, to the point that the two terms were used interchangeably by the conclusion of the study.

Daling's quantitative exploration of a possible relationship between cancer and homosexuality, prior to the outbreak of AIDS-related Kaposi's sarcoma in gay men just a few years later, necessitated a reliance on existing data sets for statistical analysis. Rather than tackle the near-impossibility of defining and quantifying homosexuality in a sample population to determine its potential causation of malignant disease, Daling used the next best available resource: two correlates of homosexuality. In their book, *Epidemiology in Medicine*, epidemiologists Charles Hennekens and Julie Buring explain, "the correlational study uses data from entire populations to compare disease frequencies between different groups during the same period of time or in the same population at different points in time."[5]

The two correlates Daling used for male homosexual behavior were a history of syphilis and never having been married. This first correlate with male homosexual behavior (syphilis) presumed, based on past case reporting, that the majority of syphilis cases involved sexual partners of the same sex. For the source of these data, the names of men diagnosed with cancer between 1974 and 1979 were matched with those in the state of Washington's syphilis registry. Second, Daling and her colleagues analyzed the records of never-married men who had participated in a National Cancer Institute study from 1973 to 1977. Like a history of syphilis infection, it was presumed that the majority of men who had never married were homosexual or had some prior same-sex sexual contact. Daling found higher rates of anal cancer in both populations: men with a past syphilis diagnosis (as compared to men who did not appear on the state syphilis registry); and men who had never married (as compared to men who had been married at some point in their lives). From these findings, the study concluded:

> We have shown that two correlates of homosexual behavior, having been recorded as reactive in a state syphilis registry and having never been married, are related to an increase in the incidence of anal cancer. Since the majority of homosexual men practice anal intercourse [citations given], the most plausible reason for these associations is that anal intercourse is a risk factor for the development of anal cancer.[6]

However, Hennekens and Buring note that, "While such correlational studies are useful for the formulation of hypotheses, they cannot be used to test them because of a number of limitations inherent in their design. Since correlational studies refer to whole populations rather than individuals, it is not possible to link an exposure to occurrence of disease in the same person."[7] Illustrating this very limitation, Daling's study does not include any data regarding how many of her subjects had indeed participated in homosexual behavior, number or frequency of sexual acts, or if anal intercourse was even part of that behavior.

Through two interweaving chains of presumptive logic and convoluted statistical correlations, associations, and relations, Daling somehow managed to assert that anal intercourse is a risk factor for anal cancer. Although the majority of Washington men who were diagnosed with syphilis in the late 1960s and early 1970s may have had same-sex sexual experiences, one cannot assume that the reverse is true: that the majority of men who have had male sexual partners have also had syphilis. Several other key caveats, although cumbersome in the mechanics of scientific journal writing's brevity, were altogether absent. These include any distinction between unprotected and protected (with a condom) anal intercourse, insertive and receptive anal practices, homosexual men and those who have only experimented with same-sex sexuality, receptive anal intercourse with or without ejaculation inside the body, monogamous or nonmonogamous sexual practices, and more. The potentially infinite laundry list of these ill-defined factors confound any correlation to a practically useless degree, and falsely reduce all same-sex sexual behavior between men to a singular, bodily act of penis-to-anus penetration.

Five years laters, in a second study published in a 1987 issue of the *New England Journal of Medicine*, Daling and nine co-authors stated with more certainty, "We conclude that homosexual behavior in men is a risk factor for anal cancer."[8] Improving upon the prior study's correlation methodology, they conducted a case-control study designed to elucidate anal cancer risk factors, including interviews, blood samples, and case controls with colon cancer who had the same disease diagnosed from 1978-1985.

Hennekens and Buring define a case-control study as, "a type of observational analytic epdemiologic investigation in which subjects are selected on the basis of whether they do (cases) or do not (controls) have a particular disease under study. The groups are then compared with respect to the proportion having a history of an exposure or characteristic of interest."[9] Advantages of case-control studies include the ability to study diseases with particularly long latency periods, require less time and resources compared to other epidemiological methods, and investigate a broader range of possible disease causation factors. As for limitations,

> The major potential problem in a case-control study relates to the fact that both the exposure and disease have already occurred at the time the participants enter into the study. As a result, the design is particularly susceptible to bias from the differential selection of either the cases or controls into the study on the basis of their exposure status as well as from differential reporting or recording of exposure information between study groups based on their disease status.[10]

To the researchers' methodological credit, interviews of subjects in this second study included questions about specific sexual practices, history of a broader range of diseases, and drug use. They found that, in men, "a history of receptive anal intercourse (related to homosexual behavior) was strongly associated with the occurrence of anal cancer."[11] The researchers admitted, however, that without a comparison group, the association between homosexuality and anal cancer results from anal intercourse, even though not all cases reported a history of this sexual act. In addition, the study's conclusion remained unsure as to whether or not anal intercourse itself was a risk factor for cancer, or rather a vehicle for some pathogen that causes anal cancer. Suspecting the latter, the study hypothesized that anal intercourse may predispose men to anal cancer by transmission of HPV or some other infection.

SMEARING THE ANUS

Despite the reductive bias and design limitations of Daling's work on cancer-causing homosexuality, the HPV-as-culprit hypothesis turned out to be a valid suspicion. In the past decade, new technologies that detect the actual presence of HPV in body tissues have established a stronger association between this viral infection and epithlelial cancers, including anal and cervical cancer. Because the most common route of HPV transmission between humans is through sexual activity, this form of cancer can theoretically be prevented by individual behavior changes, positioning the disease as an issue of concern within the domain of public health. At least two specific subtypes of the virus have a stronger statistical association with anorectal cancer than others. These are two of the four oncogenic subtypes most associated with cancers, whereas the non-ocogenic subtypes are the ones that more commonly cause genital warts.

Having substantiated this associative link between HPV and anal cancer is a far cry from determining cause and effect, however. The standard medical text *Guide to Preventive Clinical Services*, for example, states, "the natural history of how HPV infection progresses to cancer is poorly understood."[12] Joel Palefsky, a physician and medical researcher at the University of California, San Francisco who specializes in researching HPV-related anal cancer, notes, "HPV infection is likely to be necessary but insufficient for most cases of anogenital cancer," and that cofactors such as smoking, other sexually transmitted infections, oral contraceptives, and chronic irritation play a likely and important role in the development of HPV-associated diseases.[13]

Building upon the work of Daling and others in the 1980s, Palefsky has devoted a great deal of his work to an exploration of this link between HPV and malignancy, culminating in the largest body of research ever conducted on anal cancer in gay men. His findings have indicated a number of key concerns relevant to gay men's sexual health, particularly that gay men who have a history of unprotected, receptive anal intercourse are at a much higher risk for anal cancer than the average adult male. In addition, these gay men are probably at equal or higher risk for anal cancer than women, although the incidence of anal cancer is actually higher in women than men in general.

Gay men with this same history who are also HIV positive face an even greater risk than those who are HIV negative, probably due to an immune-suppressed response to HPV and cancer.[14] Until the early 1990s, the only cancers strongly associated with AIDS in gay men were Kaposi's sarcoma and non-Hodgkin's lymphoma. Recently, a noticeable increase in anal cancer has been detected in gay men with HIV, presumably because HIV-positive men are, by and large, living longer than ever before. The advent of new antiviral treatments such as protease inhibitors, aggressive treatment of opportunistic infections, and greater knowledge of preventive buttressing of the immune system have dramatically prolonged many HIV-positive gay men's lives. As these men's lifespans lengthen, there is an increasing emergence of disease that ordinarily would have taken longer to manifest than the individual's survival would have previously allowed.

BEHIND THE SCREEN

Monitoring the potential progression of anal cancer in high-risk gay men has raised a number of questions in the medical community that remain unanswered and hotly debated. Cervical cancer and anal cancer are respectively the most prevalent HPV-related cancer in women and men. Because of the strong association with HPV and the similarity of epithelial tissues involved, Palefsky and others have consistently made comparisons between anal cancer in gay men and cervical cancer in women in an attempt to demonstrate the value of implementing screening protocols. In 1994, Palefsky wrote that:

> The incidence of anal cancer in men with a history of receptive anal intercourse is probably similar to, or possibly higher than that of, cervical cancer in women before the institution of cervical cytology screening programs. Moreover, the available evidence suggests that anal cancer and its precursors are biologically similar to their cervical counterparts. Therefore, a prevention program for anal cancer similar to that for cervical cancer should be considered.[15]

That same year, a short article in the publication *AIDS Treatment News* hyped the consideration of an anal screening program:

> Unfortunately, most HIV care providers probably do not now include anal Pap smears in their daily practice. The data from studies such as Dr. Palefsky's may change that. He suggests that the following individuals should be screened annually for AIN: all HIV-infected people with CD4 counts below 500, all women with a history of high-grade CIN [cervical intraepithelial neoplasia], and all men with a history of receptive anal intercourse. Many people with these profiles may not even realize they are infected with HPV, so the monitoring should not be limited to those with a known history of anal warts.[16]

Pap smear screening may detect potentially premalignant cells and allow for timely preventive treatment, including biopsy and surgical intervention, but Palefsky's call for a widespread prevention program has frequently been met with a range of confusion, resistance, and inaction.

While the estimated incidence of anal cancer in men with a history of anal intercourse may be similar to that of women's cervical cancer before the gynecologic standardization of Pap smears, even Palefsky admits that the genesis and progression of anal cancer is poorly understood and not well-researched. Assumptions that cervical and anal cancer are similar have not been enough to convince government agencies and professional associations to adopt a protocol for anal screening, nor a consensus regarding course of action for treatment. This is exacerbated by ongoing debates surrounding the protocols for cervical Pap smear screening, which have historically defied scientific consensus in the medical literature due to a number of considerations, including the accuracy and reliability of the Pap smear, psychological impact of the smear on the patient, and cost-benefit analysis.

Critical of the unquestioned annual Pap smear for certain populations of women at lower or no risk, an editorial in the medical journal *Acta Cytologica* delved into the economic interests of a standardized procedure totaling more than a quarter of a billion dollars annual cost in the United States, stating, "Because a large volume of cervical smears is now in the hands of profit-oriented laboratory organizations, there is much vested interest in the continuation of the status quo."[17] A consensus statement published by a panel of experts participating in a National Institutes of Health conference on cervical cancer noted:

> Methods of specimen acquisition, preparation, and evaluation of the Pap smear have changed little since its introduction in the 1940s. Although it is highly effective in screening for preinvasive lesions of the cervix, a single test has a false-negative rate estimated to be 20 percent. One-half of the false negatives are due to inadequate specimen sampling, and the other half are attributed to a failure to identify the abnormal cells or to interpret them accurately.[18]

If cervical Pap smears remain tenuous after more than fifty years of clinical practice and millions of performed procedures, one can only begin to imagine the countless reasons why a recommendation for anal screening would be shot down. The September 1997 issue of San Francisco AIDS Foundation's newsletter, *Bulletin of Experimental Treatments for AIDS* (*BETA*), included a feature on HPV infection and anal disease, noting:

There are guidelines for screening and preventing ASIL in women with HIV. Although the guidelines are the subject of much debate among experts, they at least provide a blueprint. While the risks for ASIL and anal cancer are known to be increased among gay men and HIV positive women, the official word, according to the US Public Health Service (US PHS) is that 'the role of anal cytology screening (i.e., Pap smear) and treatment of ASIL in preventing anal cancer' is not well-defined. The US PHS refrains from making any recommendations whatsoever regarding periodic anal screening for detecting and treating ASIL. . . . According to Palefsky, defining target groups for screening is difficult in the absence of cost-benefit analyses that would compare the cost of anal Pap smears, coloscopies, treatment and follow-up. One reason such cost-benefit analyses have not been conducted is that the data needed to do so do not exist, creating a catch-22.[19]

Moreover, Palefsky recounted that a 1997 American Medical Association consensus conference on Pap smears briefly discussed anal screening recommendations for gay men, but concluded, "We would need a study of thousands of men" before the association would endorse a protocol, and the unlikeliness of such monumental research "dooming it."[20]

Since Palefsky made this statement about lack of cost/effectiveness measurements for anal Pap smears, one study has attempted to conduct this analysis. Researchers concluded that HIV-positive men at high risk for ASIL who receive annual Pap smears achieved significant gains in life expectancy. In addition, the cost/effectiveness ratio of annual anal Pap smears was found to be comparable to other well-accepted procedures of a preventive nature in the medical management of HIV disease.[21]

The power of the almighty "n" in quantitative research of an investigative nature has repeatedly plagued gay, lesbian, bisexual, and transgendered populations when it comes to biomedical research, as evidenced by AIDS clinical trials of pharmaceuticals, lesbian breast cancer research, sex reassignment studies, and more. The inability to recruit massive numbers of subjects from a marginalized population representing a fraction of society has come to spell disaster for a number of minority health concerns. We must ask ourselves: When a particular health concern poses an immediate threat to a specific and relatively small group of people, how do government and other approval processes that normally require studies of thousands impede the ability to generate effective prevention and treatment solutions? Direct-action activist groups such as ACT-UP have been successful in altering some of these bureaucratic systems, such as the case with the FDA's development of "fast-track" approval for drugs that show promise in treating AIDS.[22] Can or should similar systems be established for the adoption of protocols, technologies, and procedures such as anal Pap smears? Chapters 2 and 3 in this book point to the ongoing escalation of this problem and how the sometimes unflexible standards of quantitative rigor can exacerbate problems that defy traditional public health approaches.

While the Pap smear procedure has been charged with ethical and technical debate related to epithelial cancers, it is only one component of effective screening. A complex process of examination, biopsy, and cytology are also usually necessary to determine the course of treatment action, if any. Visual identification of lesions with a colposcope is especially important. Traditionally inserted into the vagina, the colposcope is a viewing device used to illuminate and magnify tissue inside the body. Gynecologists frequently use colposcopes to locate cervical lesions in the case of an abnormal pap smear. Colposcopy is also important for anal surveillance because, without magnification, the medical examiner might not be able to detect the flat lesions embedded in the tissue, even with the application of acetic acid, which will render many lesions visible. While the colposcope is valuable because it can be used to locate internal lesions in the case of an abnormal pap smear result, it is an expensive piece of equipment that is often not readily available outside of gynecologic practices, especially for the anal examination of a male.

Access to colposcopy is but one complication in the gender confusion provoked by anal Pap smears for men. As demonstrated by my own smear experience, the performance of the traditionally female procedure on a male patient throws a wrench into the complex biomedical machinery of standardized practice and professional specialization. Take, for example, Palefsky's body of work. Leading the scientific investigation of anal Pap smears, Palefsky's research clinic at the University of California San Francisco Hospital remains situated within their Department of Gynecology, despite their ongoing clinical studies comprised of predominantly male subjects. This points to a larger structural problem within social and organizational development as it currently exists: the virtual absence of a men's health social movement and the lack of attention to gay male health within medical and social practice. Whereas the field of gynecology has emerged in recent decades to address the necessary specialization in women's reproductive and sexual health, there is no comparable, comprehensive approach to a male equivalent.

In the case of anal cancer, the problems associated with a lack of integrated approaches to men's health exceed the need for preventive screening. When a smear detects abnormal cells in anal tissue that *could* progress to cancer, the decision to surgically intervene is a tenuous one fraught with both ethical and logistical complications, for " . . . there have been no formal treatment trials comparing different methods of therapy to prove that treatment of AIN [anal intraepithelial neoplasia] prevents cancer."[23] Palefsky has explained how this creates a frustrating situation for referring male patients. A practically identical lesion would be easily and quickly treated if detected on the cervix, but not the anal canal. In a presentation at the 1997 National Lesbian and Gay Health Association conference, Palefsky speculated, "You might find an enlightened gynecologist who would be willing to see a male for an anal HPV evaluation." He noted the prevalence of homophobia among anal surgeons as one of the most significant barriers to accessing early treatment for lesions before they have the chance to progress to a dangerous state.

Despite the combined emergence and professional notice of potentially beneficial screening techniques applicable to male bodies, the male specificity of prostate cancer, men's sexual health concerns, and so on, there has been no serious consideration of an established field of medical specialization for men's health, nor male sexual health in particular. An often disjointed combination of general practice, proctology, urology, internal medicine, and a number of other specializations has been utilized instead. Over time, the health and wellness of female bodies have coalesced into a gender-specific medical practice and field of research, whereas the care and inquiry of male bodies have been organized along differing lines of social categories that are usually not directly related to gender and biological sex.

The historical treatment of women as being inherently diseased has been well-documented, as has the placement of women as an objectified other to be studied under the medical and male gaze. While gay men have been subjected to similar forms of medicalization, there remain a number of differences between women and gay men in these power relations bound up with gender, sex, and sexuality as they are structured by medical science as a cultural and social practice. In her book *Public Privates: Performing Gynecology from Both Ends of the Speculum*, Terri Kapsalis defines gynecology as the "quintessential examination of women. Gynecology is not simply the study of women's bodies—gynecology makes female bodies. It defines and constitutes female bodies. . . . In gynecology's many and varied practices and representations are found condensations of cultural attitudes and anxieties about women, female bodies, and female sexualities."[24] There is no male equivalent of a medical site that constitutes male bodies and sexualities in such a localized way. Perhaps this is one reason for gay men's historical inability to organize a truly revolutionary approach to redefining health care similar to the work of women's health movements. The zones of contestation are more fragmented and less condensed within medicine due to the nature of how those zones have been constructed by the prevalence of male privilege from within the profession of medicine. Through new formulations of medical technology, some male bodies and anal sexualities have been subsumed under the valence of gynecology, demanding a renewed analysis of how gay men are affected by women's health treatment.

COMPARATIVE SEX

The logic of an analogous approach to both cervical and anal cancers relies in part on common sense, while at the same time risks a degree of problematic assumption. As body sites for receptive sexual penetration, the vagina and rectum have been consistently compared by medical scientists since the early 1980s as entry points for HIV infection. Cultural theorists such as Cindy Patton, Leo Bersani, and Paula Treichler have examined the processes and implications of such comparison over time.[25] Often framed by medical science as reservoirs of contagion, the sexualized anatomy of the two areas have now become zones for heightened scrutiny of cancerous development. In the case of HPV-related cancer, this comparison has narrowed and localized from the vagina/rectum to the cervix/anus. As the medical newsletter *BETA* explains:

> Squamous epithelial tissue forms the skin and the linings of the mouth, pharynx (throat), esophagus, lower vagina and anus. Columnar epithelium lines the digestive tract from the stomach to the anal canal, and most of the uterus. In the lower portion of the uterus called the cervix and inside the anal canal, the tissue types meet and overlap. Although HPV may infect any site in the squamous epithelium, it most often infects these vulnerable transitional zones and causes lesions. Most cases of cervical or anal cancer also develop in these regions.[26]

The combination of these similarities, both in the epithelium as well as the epidemiological prevalence of HPV in those who practice receptive sexual intercourse, has juxtaposed the two anatomic locales as sites for preventive intervention and heightened surveillance.

Cultural theorist Catherine Waldby has described medicine's analogizing of heterosexual women and homosexual men as receptive sexual partners in relation to disease by stating, "The bodies of gay and bisexual men and women are considered to be implicated in the spread of infection because of their inherent permeability. They are imagined to form fluid, infectious circuits and ambiguous relationships with other bodies, either sexual or uterine."[27] Leo Bersani has discussed the popular vilification of receptivity and penetrability in epidemic moments, commenting on the popular imagination that women and gay men become hungry reservoirs seeking out sexual contagion. While the Pap smear may be a screening technology in the sense that it is a procedure for collecting epithelial cells from a body, preserving them, and conducting a cytological analysis, it also functions as a social and cultural technology to construct the patient's history, present state of being, and future.

Women who receive abnormal Pap smears, indicating the detection of cells that could be precancerous, often report experiencing a sense of shame and self-blame in the diagnosis of what could be disease. The uncertainty of abnormality and the ambiguity of potentially precancerous results leave many patients with anxiety about their present and future health status, in part because they are unable to read their own bodies without the assistance and interpretation of medical science. Tina Posner has written of this moment when a new dependence is created, citing the damage that may emerge when the relationships between medical technology, clinician, and patient form an unhealthy reliance:

> In cervical cytology screening, medical assertion of the significance of a sign unavailable to women is an attempt to control uncertain future developments—to extend clinical control over risk. In the absence of acknowledgment of the uncertainty and a fuller sharing of information and language, which could allow a discussion of the risks of intervention or nonintervention, medical aims prevail. Women's health status is defined for them in a way that is disempowering and unhealthy.[28]

The abnormality of a cancer screening should not be understated. Not only does the diagnosis reside in a zone of gray interpretation and multiple possibilities for outcome, it can be a defining moment that collides with one's self-identity and measure by others. In a study of women's reactions to receiving an abnormal Pap smear diagnosis, medical sociologist Shireem Rajaram has attempted to make sense of how this particular medical diagnosis constructs social and cultural meaning for the patient.

> . . . the diagnosis of an abnormal Pap smear is more than just a practical adaptation to the physical demands of the diagnosis or illness. It is a process through which the self is negotiated, maintained, and expressed through the medium of the illness within the context of everyday life. The underlying driving force is to maintain one's moral worth in the public domain.[29]

The fact that the abnormality may be in some way related to their sexual history magnifies the experience, indicative of the questionable "moral worth" Rajaram writes about. Tina Posner has also explored the power relations that are constituted at the time of diagnosis, observing,

> Aetiological factors relating to contraceptive use and the male partner's sexual history or occupation have not been given so much attention as the woman's sexual history. The result for women with abnormal Pap smears may be that they come to feel highly embarrassed because of the implied guilt—the stigma of having an abnormal smear, and that their own versions of their bodily history are discounted.[30]

Selective application of the smear to specific bodies is an additional concern within the context of disempowerment and moral measurement, for the Pap smear is usually not a one-time event. The frequency of the smear is often calculated by the degree to which one meets the stigmatized definition of high-risk. Take, for example, the following recommendation excerpted from a medical text that attempts to discern the criteria for frequency of screening:

> It seems reasonable to assume that the socially stable woman with limited sexual exposure who had three prior negative smears is at an extremely low risk of developing cervical cancer and could be safely screened every second or third year. It seems equally reasonable to assume that a socially unstable, promiscuous woman should continue to have annual screenings.[31]

The factors of social unstability (however that gets defined) and promiscuity (also a problematic term) thus become the yardsticks of repeated screening. Similar criteria have been suggested in the past for periodic HIV-antibody testing, relying upon the faulty logic of characterizing the individual as a member of a high-risk group rather than concentrating on the specific behavior and detailed life history that places an individual at risk.

Now that Pap smears are used on gay male bodies for similar purposes of HPV-related cancer screening, how might gay men's sense of identity, body image, public worth, and overall state of health be affected? How might we prevent a smearing of the queer so as not to repeat gynecology's historical disempowerment of women? It is useful to conduct some comparative analyses of the social stigmas attached to the illnesses of anal cancer in gay men, cervical cancer in women, HPV, and AIDS in an attempt to understand exactly what is at stake for gay men as the controversies of anal Pap screening continue to unfold. Philosopher Susan Sontag explores the historical differences and similarities between cancer and sexually transmitted infection, particularly AIDS. She notes a distinction of meanings in cancer and AIDS that are embedded in the genesis of the illness—namely, how it came to be acquired:

> Because of countless metaphoric flourishes that have made cancer synonymous with evil, having cancer has been experienced by many as shameful, therefore something to conceal, and also unjust, a betrayal of one's body. Why me? the cancer patient exclaims bitterly. With AIDS, the shame is linked to an imputation of guilt; and the scandal is not at all obscure.[32]

Sontag further explains that, "The sexual transmission of this illness, considered by most people as a calamity one brings on oneself, is judged more harshly than other means—especially since AIDS is understood as a disease not only of sexual excess but of perversity."[33] Historically, cancer was not thought to be a product of viral infection, but the differences between the two have now become quite blurred. The recent determination that Kaposi's sarcoma is most likely caused by a form of herpes virus is an excellent example of this. Gay men's anal cancer, caused predominantly by sexually transmitted HPV infection, smears the two phenomenon that Sontag seeks to contrast in her analysis. The illnesses of cancer and sexually transmitted infection are no longer distinct; they have become juxtaposed in a unique hybrid of dense social, cultural, and scientific metaphor.

The possible implications for this hybridized stigma are numerous. Sontag states with full confidence that "Infectious diseases to which sexual fault is attached always inspire fears of easy contagion and bizarre fantasies of transmission by nonvenereal means in public places."[34] This irrationality of the popular imagination has, time and again, lent itself to public health measures that restrict the rights of individuals based on fear rather than available information, usually for the stated good of the general population. Lest we stand by and witness gay men's anal cancer become yet another illness used to politically mobilize the systemic denial of human rights (as has been the case with gay bowel syndrome, which I discussed earlier in this book), the need to frame HPV-related cancers in nonprejudicial ways should be painfully clear.

Take, for example, a piece of proposed legislation authored by Oklahoma congressman and obstetrician Tom Coburn. In his justification for the "HIV Prevention Act of 1997," Coburn has cited HPV-related anal cancer as one of many reasons to enact the bill, which would effectively abolish anonymous HIV testing, impose mandatory HIV testing on pregnant women, mandate contact tracing of sexual partners who may have been exposed to HIV, and more. As recognition of anal cancer prevalence in gay male and female populations grows within the medical community and extends into more popular discourse, we find ourselves in the unique position of being presently afforded the opportunity to influence the values attached to this epidemiology *as* it takes shape, rather than wishing in hindsight that we had denounced the inappropriateness and inaccuracy of sexual vilification before it solidified (as was the early 1980s case with GRID).

NEGOTIATING THE SMEAR

I have had an annual anal Pap smear since 1995, and will continue to do so. Fortunately, I have health insurance and access to a competent and sensitive physician. Many gay men are not so privileged. As an assertive health consumer, I've assessed my own sexual history and determined that I am, in fact, at some risk for anal cancer. Although probably not at high risk, the Pap smear remains an important preventive component of my ongoing health care, and I intend to utilize the technology at my and my physician's disposal. I am acutely aware, however, of the social circumstances I endure as the result of this choice. When I received the results from my first Pap smear indicating mild dysplasia, my first reaction was to make sense of the experience in relation to my sexual identity, past behaviors, and current lifestyle—all through a lens of negativity and self-blame. The smearing occurred on a number of planes beyond that of microbiology, including even the blurred boundaries of my own gender identity as coded in my clinical computer profile and beyond. There exists a gaping void in the psychological, social, and cultural implications of the anal smear, and much research is needed to determine the qualitative effects such smearing has on gay male patients.

If Pap smears are to be negotiated on an even playing field of power relations between patient and provider, lab technician and lay consumer, and scientist and research subject, a great deal of work is at hand. How can activists, clinicians, health organizations, and others foster a more democratic form of biomedical science and protocol implementation that enable gay men to define their health status in collaboration with the fields of medicine and policy making? Although gay men's rates of anal cancer might not currently be so high as to warrant routine, widespread screening, the increasing lifespan of gay men with HIV will necessitate closer monitoring of emergent cancerous trends. In comparison, rates of anal cancer are higher among gay and bisexual men than rates of cervical cancer in women.[35] This involves the development of screening recommendations that do not set into motion a practice of epidemiological surveillance and treatment control that further stigmatize and pathologize gay male sexuality and anal pleasure.

Learning a lesson from feminist critiques of clinical Pap smear experiences, how do we screen for gay men's anal cancer without inscribing upon them a sense of defilement, invasion, disempowerment, and blame? This challenge serves as another example of how gay men could greatly benefit from the knowledge and progress produced by women's health movements.[36] As evidenced by the other chapters in this book that are devoted to topical microbicides and internal condoms, the health of women and gay men have become inextricably linked as sexual practices and sexually transmitted infections are increasingly mediated and regulated by technological means. Effective strategizing and advocacy in this domain will necessitate women and gay men's increased cross-participation in each others' health activism and the formation of collaborative social movements for the achievement of mutually successful ends.

Adviser

One day in class
I politely asked,
"If queer boys' greatest risk
is each other's fluids,
why not tie off some cord
or somesuchthing
to keep them from flowing?"
I wondered.

And my dyke professor
replied that it's just easier
for them to wear condoms.
But how could she know
the heat and fear
between men?
I wondered.

Later I decided to read
her dissertation on bodies.
In the introduction it's '81.
While living in the Castro,
working in the typing pool,
home one day with a bottle
of beer and a newspaper,
she read about gay cancer.
Looking at a mark on her skin,
she wondered.

I remembered our talk
about my thesis
during office hours
when she asked me
how much time I had
planned to finish
and I wondered.

Chapter 5

Something Borrowed, Something Blue: Viagra Use Among Gay Men

The drug sildenafil citrate was approved by the Food and Drug Administration on March 27, 1998, under the brand name Viagra, for the treatment of male erectile dysfunction, more commonly referred to as impotence. Viagra, patented and sold by the pharmaceutical company Pfizer, quickly became the fastest-selling drug in American medical history and has been heralded in popular media as a pill that could revolutionize men's sexual relationships with women. In its first four months on the market, demand for Viagra in the United States exceeded 1.5 million prescriptions, and the drug has been forecast to reach one billion dollars in sales during its first year.[1]

After its initial few months of booming sales, consumption of Viagra slowed considerably, with the rate of new prescriptions decreased to approximately one-half.[2] A number of factors are responsible for this tapering off, chiefly because the drug is usually not covered by insurance companies and costs about $10 per pill, Viagra does not always eliminate impotence, and it sometimes causes undesirable side effects such as headaches, nausea, and blue-tinted vision. Large numbers of men also quickly realized they had been misled by popular accounts of the drug's aphrodisiac effects. It does not directly induce a spontaneous erection, nor does it create the rabid libido that has become part of the urban mythology surrounding this drug. Viagra simply increases the flow of blood to the pelvic area. In combination with sexual arousal, this facilitates achieving and maintaining an erection in some men who have had previous difficulty with "getting it up." In affect, if you are not already turned on by your sex partner, your fantasy, or your hand, Viagra won't do it for you.

In addition, not all cases of impotence result from physiological impairment; psychological conditions such as depression and anxiety can also be causes. Other men realized that the cost of each Viagra pill, which comes in 25, 50, and 100 mg tablets, cost the same no matter which dose is prescribed. Some men ask their physician for a 100 mg dose and then cut each tablet in half, reducing the cost of their prescription by fifty percent. Because of Pfizer's heavy marketing efforts, many men continued to receive free samples from their physician for occasional use rather than paying for a prescription.

The marked decrease in Viagra use coincided with an array of news reports that collectively cast a shadow on the drug's success story. Soon thereafter, the FDA posted a summary of cases documenting that sixty-nine Americans taking Viagra had died between late March and July 1998, with forty-six of the deaths linked to cardiovascular incidents. A widow in California, for example, announced she was planning to sue Pfizer because her sixty-five-year-old husband collapsed and died after taking the drug and engaging in sexual activity.[3]

These concerns soon extended into gay communities as anecdotal reports began to circulate about gay men who had died using Viagra in conjunction with "poppers." Formerly known as amyl nitrate, poppers are a commonly used recreational drug, inhaled by some gay men to enhance sexual experience. A combination of the two substances can cause a life-threatening drop in blood pressure. Initial concerns included the potential for dangerous side effects from the combination of Viagra and certain protease inhibitors used for HIV antiviral therapy. The latter speculation proved insubstantial, however. In an article published in the *Bay Area Reporter,* Doctors Herminia Palacio and Mitchell Katz of the San Francisco Department of Public Health advised that ". . . Viagra will cause a small temporary increase in the blood levels of protease inhibitors (which does not lead to resistance and is unlikely to produce side effects.) Therefore no change in the dose of protease inhibitors in recommended."[4]

In a rare move by a pharmaceutical company, Pfizer approached the Gay and Lesbian Medical Association (GLMA) about their concerns with these interactions. Ben Schatz, executive director for GLMA, noted that it spoke well for Pfizer, saying, "Imagine a pharmaceutical company approaching a gay and lesbian medical group about something not HIV related. On that level what they did is really important and should be applauded."[5] Shortly after that meeting between the two organizations, GLMA issued a press release to gay and mainstream media that outlined precautions with points of consideration for physicians prescribing Viagra, their patients, and the gay community at large. Among other things, the organization recommended that, "Medical providers and patients should discuss all recreational drug use, especially the use of 'poppers' or other forms of inhaled nitrates, prior to prescribing Viagra."[6]

In a classic case of the clash between gay cultural norms and government health regulation, Pfizer spokesperson Maryann Caprino told *The New York Times* how their efforts to issue early warnings about the dangers of Viagra and the use of poppers in gay male communities were hindered:

> "We want people to make the connection between nitrates and poppers," Ms. Caprino said. She said the warning about nitrates appears in Viagra's Federally approved package insert. But, she said, "You can't use words like 'poppers' in your insert." And sales representatives making the rounds to New York doctors in the last two weeks "could only talk off the package insert," she said, which meant they couldn't use the word poppers either.[7]

To their credit, the staff of Pfizer submitted new educational materials for Federal approval that would spell out poppers loud and clear. The lack of forethought given to this complication, combined with a bureaucratic system that impedes quick and easy adaptation for culturally specific market education, does not bode well for future health technologies with the potential to create even more severe problems.

On July 12, 1998, the news wire service United Press International distributed an article in which the mayor of West Hollywood, a community largely populated with gay men, issued a public statement to educate local men about these dangers. Mayor Steve White stated several men had died from using Viagra along with crystal methamphetamine.

One of the long-term benefits to AIDS organizing has been the establishment of relatively rapid and effective response networks of health organizations, gay medical professionals, and open lines of communication to the private sector in the face of an emerging health concern. In San Francisco, activist and scholar Eric Rofes had already pitched an idea for a town hall meeting on gay men's use of Viagra to Stop AIDS Project, a nonprofit HIV education and prevention organization. I served as a panelist for the discussion along with Rofes and Boston's Fenway Health Center physician Marshall Forstein. Timing of the discussion was well-planned and became incorporated into a larger track of workshops on gay men's sexual cultures that took place during the National Lesbian and Gay Health Association's annual conference.

In a workshop that had taken place earlier in the health conference, I presented some of my work on gay men's access to a number of sexual technologies, several of which are the topics of chapters in this book, including the female condom for anal sex, Pap smears to screen for anal cancer in men who practice receptive anal intercourse, and rectal microbicides as a form of condomless chemical barrier for safer sex. At the suggestion of a colleague, I approached a physician at the conference and asked for a Viagra prescription so that I might try the drug myself before speaking about it a few nights later. Getting hard has never really been a problem for me, but I was curious to know why so many gay men who are not impotent are raving about its effects. Let's just say I was quite pleased with the noticeable results myself.

In preparing my remarks for the panel on gay men's use of Viagra, it occurred to me that the drug had become the latest episode in gay men's appropriation of technologies, heterosexist in their design and marketing, for officially unsanctioned use. The Viagra brochure that is published and distributed by Pfizer, for example, includes text that is heterosexist in its narrative, complete with photos depicting a middle-to-upper-class straight couple who are white, look to be well over the age of fifty, and in a long-term relationship. Some of the hypothetical patient concerns resolved by the brochure include:

Will my partner know how much I desire her, or will she think my erection is just due to the medication?

We've let other things—our jobs, the kids—take over our lives. I'm not sure how to get our love life started again.[8]

In addition to Pfizer's marketing materials, much of the media hype surrounding Viagra has concentrated predominantly on older heterosexual couples, with seventy-four-year old, failed U.S. Presidential candidate Bob Dole becoming one of their unofficial spokespersons. In one public statement, he said, "It's a great drug. I wish I'd bought stock earlier."[9]

Results of the first prospective study of erectile dysfunction in gay men were announced in August 1998 by researcher Leslie Goldberg at the World Meeting on Impotence Research in Amsterdam, demonstrating gay men's need for access to such treatments. Data were collected from 460 gay men who had responded to questionnaires distributed in the Castro neighborhood of San Francisco. Researchers were able to determine that approximately seven percent of the men reported having experienced erectile dysfunction that was psychologically based, and six percent reported having experienced dysfunction that was organically based.[10] Psychologically based erectile dysfunction was also found to be significantly higher in HIV-positive men.

RECREATIONAL ERECTIONS

While certainly some gay men use Viagra to alleviate problems associated with impotence, many others use the drug as an enhancement of otherwise normal sexual functioning. As recognition of gay men's and others' recreational use of Viagra grew, public opinions condemning nonmedical use of the drug were quickly fashioned in a timely response. In an editorial titled "Society Abusing Medical Marvel," the Ft. Lauderdale newspaper *Sun-Sentinel* comments,

The medical community can do a much better job of curbing this form of ignorance and pharmaceutical abuse. Physicians, health care, and Medicaid officials must make sure Viagra reaches those individuals who have a bonafide case of erectile dysfunction, and not to men simply seeking a good time.

If not, Viagra will continue to be the butt of late night TV monologues, the subject of questionable public policy and an abused medication that once offered so much promise.[11]

The editorial's concern with recreational use of Viagra seems to be much more social than pharmaceutical, worried about the growing stigma, jabbing humor, and economic drain attached to the drug rather than the potential for widespread body harm. The line of distinction here is rather rigid: Viagra should be used only by men with a serious impairment, and recreational use of the drug to further enhance sexual ability creates a needless and damaging hedonism that attracts mockery in its excess. In other words, don't ruin it for the rest of us.

At least one research group on drug policy is advocating that Viagra be placed on the Federal Government's list of controlled substances. Michael T. Risher, who is the legal affairs adviser for the Lindesmith Center, argued in an opinion column published in *The New York Times* that:

> For men with serious impotence problems, like those who have had prostate surgery, it may be the best way ever for them to have a "normal" sex life or bear children. But many men—both the 70-year-olds who want to regain part of their lost youth and the 25-year-olds who want to enhance their sexual performance—are simply interested in purchasing the ability to have more sex. This nonmedical use of a substance is what the law considers abuse.[12]

But Risher fails to make a convincing argument, admitting the drug is relatively safe while offering an uncompelling and vague warning that "long-term health effects are unknown." In addition, Viagra is nonaddictive, unlike many narcotics and other drugs on the controlled substance list that prohibits physicians from prescribing them for nonmedical reasons. Risher never specifies which law considers "purchasing the ability to have more sex" as abusive, nor does he outline what the inherent dangers of more sex might be. He also fails to define what a normal sex life should be, and for whom, although clearly procreation is a legitimate component within this realm.

The construction of a normative male sexuality also exempts homosexuality, either explicitly or implicitly, as healthy sex is discussed only within the context of fertilization and rejuvenation of established, heterosexual relationships. In the Annapolis, Maryland, newspaper *The Capital*, Peter H. Gott writes an advice column answering readers' health-related questions. After suggesting to an unmarried, impotent man that he consult his physician about Viagra as a solution to his erectile woes, one angry reader felt the need to respond, saying, "If he were unmarried or homosexual, he shouldn't be prescribed Viagra or any other product to assist him. In such an instance, he should remain celibate and should not even masturbate. Rather, he must obtain counseling from the church, because moral guidance is the option preferred by our Creator."[13] In a tiresome rehash of imposed Christian morality, the respondent gives an imperative that commonly crops up in debates surrounding Viagra and other health technologies. In this case, it is the argument that the drug should only be used to assist nature and the creator of nature's will.

Clearly, some people feel that Viagra should be limited to impotent men who possess specific characteristics and only engage in a narrowly defined set of sexual acts. Aside from gay men's recreational use of the drug, a range of other uses deemed illegitimate or unintended have also drawn the attention of the popular and mass media. The mayor of Bocaiuva do Sul in Brazil doled out free supplies of the drug in hopes that it would boost his town's population, thereby increasing funding from his country's federal government. Some zoologists and veterinarians are hoping the drug can be utilized to produce results similar in animals, for breeding purposes. Many women have begun taking Viagra with the belief that it improves genital blood flow and might help to promote their sexual arousal as well, even though the drug has not been officially approved or well tested for female bodies.[14] Viagra is clearly one of those cases in which technology has outpaced public policy, and the long-term social impact of this and other impotence treatments has yet to be realized.

SEX AS A CLASS ACT

Because Viagra was approved for use in the United States more than six months before its approval in Britain, the hype surrounding the drug in the U.S. media served as something of an omen for the United Kingdom. The expected British stampede for the drug has raised endless doubt and speculation overseas about the potential for economic burden to be shouldered by European governments' health programs. One English newspaper reported:

> [General Practitioners] announced at a recent British Medical Association meeting that they feared the drug could place a pounds 1 billion burden on their budgets. Health Minister Alan Milburn has tried to assuage their worries by insisting it would only be prescribed to patients with a legitimate medical case.[15]

Britain's National Health Service eventually decided to provide Viagra to gay men once it became available through the government health care system, despite outcries from such organizations as the Conservative Family Institute and Family and Youth Concern.

An Irish physician warned that once Viagra became available in his country, demand for the drug would break the health service, stating, "If this is offered free to a man on the dole and is costing pounds five a time, that could mean the taxpayer is paying up to pounds 35 a week to support this unemployed man's sex life. To make it worse, we'll have to pick up the bill for any children born as a result of his endeavours."[16] In a time of international backlash against welfare systems, Viagra raises the ugly prospect in conservative imaginations of an impoverished population explosion. In this unlikely scenario, both the sex that spawned the children and the offspring themselves are subsidized by state dollars, truly welfare babies from the very moment of conception.

In the United States, debates continue as to whether or not forms of public assistance such as Medicaid or private insurance will pick up the tab or pay a percentage of Viagra prescriptions. Most HMOs do not cover Viagra, while some ration payment to men for eight pills a month. Interestingly, other pharmaceutical treatments such as Caverject, which is injected directly into the base of the penis to induce an erection, is more frequently covered by insurance companies. The company that produces Caverject, Pharmacia and Up-john, recommends using the injection no more than three times a week. Pfizer, in comparison, recommends using Viagra no more than every twenty-four hours.[17] By design, Viagra possesses the potential for great consumption due to its rate of use.

The emerging sexual technologies discussed in this book represent a growing trend in the enablement of safer and healthy sexual activity in that these accessories are increasingly defined by their market potential and profitability. Upon its introduction for over-the-counter sale, for example, Reality female condoms cost approximately three dollars apiece. Polyurethane condoms in the traditional design of a sheath worn on the penis sell for as much as ten times their latex counterparts. Viagra tablets sell for ten dollars each (and two to three times that amount on the black market). Factor in lubricant that costs an average of more than a dollar per ounce, and one can easily imagine how personal finances could quickly dictate the amount and kind of sex for individuals with even an average libido. While latex condoms remain relatively inexpensive and are often distributed at no cost by community public health organizations, the prospect of technological sex stratified by class already exists.

CRIMINAL AIDS AND CRIMINAL AIDS

While society at large may recognize impotence treatments for men as a breakthrough of medical marvel, public policymakers have encountered a host of ethical and political quandaries in regulating access to substances that could perpetuate sexual activity deemed unhealthy, dangerous, and even criminal. Sexually active individuals in two categories have posed the most pressing debates concerning how access to Viagra should be restricted or granted: men who have tested HIV positive and men who have been classified as sex offenders.

The importance of Viagra in the lives of HIV-positive men may be considerable given the psychological and physiological stress accompanying HIV disease and its treatments. These same stressors can contribute to impotence, complicating sexual activity for sero-positive men far beyond the anxieties associated with transmission and stigma. Additionally, the relative success of protease inhibitors has not been without a number of undesirable side effects. While diarrhea, kidney stones, and fatty deposits nicknamed protease paunch may be reported in the media, the impotence associated with antiretroviral combination therapy has gone largely unexamined as worthy of address in popular and medical literature. In a column for *POZ* magazine, writer Greg Lugliani lamented, "Like many positive guys, what kept me limp is what keeps me alive—my antiretroviral cocktail."[18] The arrival of Viagra, however, has revolutionized Lugliani's sex life (or lack thereof) in a way that hormones and other treatment attempts had miserably failed.

It should come as no surprise that some conservative elements might view the capability of HIV-positive men to become sexually active as akin to a loaded gun, encouraging the transmission of HIV by means of libidinous pharmacology. Take, for example, the many Veteran's Affairs (VA) hospitals across the United States that have prohibited their doctors from prescribing Viagra. Even some VA medical center pharmacies, such as the one in Fresno, will not fill a prescription for Viagra even if prescribed by an outside, private physician. In late 1998, the Veteran's Affairs Washington headquarters commissioned a national panel to evaluate safety and ethical issues surrounding Viagra, including whether or not it should be made available to men who are HIV positive or known to be sex offenders.

In *The Fresno Bee,* Pfizer spokesperson Pam Gemmel agreed that "the drug shouldn't go to men who have been convicted of a sex crime," while Fresno VA spokesperson David Phillips was quoted as stating, "It still needs to be determined whether a doctor could ask about a patient's criminal history."[19] The definitional status of sex offender and the criminal nature of specific sexual acts will undoubtedly have bearing on gay men throughout the country who have been convicted of crimes related to consensual public sex and sodomy, among other practices.

Beyond the establishment of restrictive policies for Viagra, the possibility of punitive legal measures to hold physicians responsible for distribution of Viagra to "dangerous" men has already been discussed. Republican state representative Larry Sims had announced that if he was reelected to office in 1998, he intended to introduce state legislation criminalizing the prescription of Viagra to men who are known to be HIV positive. Reminding us that he is a former nurse, Sims attempts to speak with both medical and government authority in his bid to regulate private sexual activity under the auspices of unsound epidemiological speculation. The idea stemmed from his statements that he was reasonably sure that he know of a physician prescribing Viagra to a man with HIV, which he deems "gross malpractice."[20] He argues that Viagra should be withheld from men who are HIV positive lest physicians usher in a new wave of sexually rampant Typhoid Marys who would fan the flames of the epidemic. His proposal is not limited to Viagra and HIV, but also includes "any other sexual aid to a person with a known sexually transmitted disease."[21]

CONVERSION THERAPY: BOTTOMS BECOME TOPS

Viagra is clearly beginning to have an impact on the social and behavioral roles of "tops" and "bottoms" within gay male communities. While not mutually exclusive, many gay men self-identify as being primarily a top (the insertive partner in penetrative anal sex), bottom (the receptive partner who is penetrated), or versatile. Some tops who have developed problems achieving and maintaining erections due to factors such as age or HIV treatment, for example, may no longer be able to get hard enough to participate in anal sex. Some of these tops have reported that in order for them to continue to participate in the meaningful act of anal intercourse, they have chosen to take on the role of bottom rather than abstain from the practice altogether. Such was the case with one man who attended the town hall meeting on gay men's Viagra use in San Francisco. During the discussion portion of the program, he stated that ever since he was prescribed Viagra, he no longer *had* to be the bottom—not out of force, but by default. In his column for *POZ* magazine, Greg Lugliani recalls, ". . . this once-proud top tried his best to be a better bottom."[22]

With the exception of this conversion therapy of bottoms into tops, a disturbing trend in the flood of discourse surrounding Viagra and gay men has been the nearly exclusive focus of attention on the top. Relegation to the role of bottom can generate a great deal of sympathy, especially knowing the ways in which bottoms are frequently devalued in most gay male cultures as less masculine, less desirable, and somehow weak in their almost feminine-like submission to sexual penetration.[23] Other than the obvious benefits Viagra provides to tops, how might the drug alter the sex lives of men who are primarily bottoms? We know that Viagra increases blood flow to the genital region, but so far, public discussion in the gay media has focused on the penis. From personal experience, I discovered that Viagra can also create a marked increase in pleasurable anal sensation for the bottom. The enhancement of receptive anal intercourse should also warrant closer study by both medical and social scientists.

One theoretical health concern for gay male bottoms using Viagra might be an increased susceptibility for infection by sexually transmitted agents. Warnings about the use of poppers includes a theory that nitrates could facilitate the transmission of pathogens beyond the outer rectal lining and into the bloodstream. A public health education brochure targeting gay men titled *Poppers: Can You Afford the Risk?* asserts that, "Dilated blood vessels in the rectum caused by sniffing poppers make it easier for viruses and other germs to enter your bloodstream. If you sniff poppers and your partner cums in you, you're wide open for infection."[24] If Viagra has a similar effect of dilation and increased blood flow in the pelvic area, this could place him more at risk. Simultaneously, if rectal tearing results in heavier bleeding because of this dilation, the top may be exposed to more risk as well.

The phenomenon of Viagra's conversion of bottoms into tops has been heralded more in terms of impending doom than a form of sexual liberation, however. In the latest of a series of attacks on gay male circuit parties and recreational drug use, journalist Gabriel Rotello continued his sensational predictions of a new wave of infections that hearken back to the early 1980s. In his one-page opinion column published in *The Advocate*, Rotello surmises,

> It is precisely among drug abusers that Viagra's potential for harm looms largest. Crystal meth in particular makes its users sexually voracious but impotent—a world of bottoms searching for a top. The epidemiological effect of a drug that, in the

words of one crystal user, "turns every bottom into a top as well," could really give HIV transmission a nasty boost.[25]

In the same column, Rotello also quotes a physician friend who feared Viagra was likely to "throw gasoline on the gay sexual revolution."

A rehash of his Chicken Little routine, Rotello introduces some interesting scenarios, yet it remains impossible to predict the likelihood of Viagra's impact, if any, on HIV seroprevalence in gay male populations. While some unsafe bottoms will become unsafe tops, yet other men who have had problems keeping it up while wearing a condom may now be able to get and stay hard using protection like never before. The likely outcome will be that epidemiologists will invest neither the time nor the money in tracing any single drug's influence on safer sex practices and disease transmission to the degree that such a pinpointed calculation could be made on any large scale.

HOW HARD IS HARD ENOUGH?

The meaning of the phallus remains somewhat underexplored in gay male culture, with respect to why a stiff penis should be the predominant focus of gay male sexuality. For many gay men, an erection is not always the center or most desirable component of sex—in watersports for example, an erection can actually hinder the sexual act at hand. In some ways, the introduction of Viagra as a sexual technology in gay men's sex reinforces an unfortunate drive to achieve one of the ideals of hypermasculine perfection—the ability to always be able to become erect, to get very hard (what Dr. Marshall Forstein calls the hardness of "a seventeen-year-old's erection"), and to stay that way indefinitely. Whereas sometimes reality intervened to make this a near-impossibility, Viagra and its pharmaceutical counterparts (such as Caverject) offer a scientific means to mythical ends. Viagra has already become a standard prop on the sets of gay male porn production, ensuring viewers will no longer have to see video footage and photos of unsightly limpness, unless (in some rare cases) that is what the producer intended to depict.

But just how hard is hard enough? In drug testing and development, clinical trials attempt to measure erectile success along a spectrum from flaccid to fully erect. As with a great deal of scientific research on sexual technologies, this method of measurement is immensely, if not exclusively, heterosexist in its very definition. In one study of Caverject published in the *International Journal of Impotence Research*, "Optimal response was defined as erection sufficient to permit vaginal penetration and lasting 30 to 60 minutes."[26] Another study in the *Journal of Urology* measures erectile success in terms of "patient and spouse satisfaction" and concluded one medication ". . . was highly effective at producing penile rigidity and an erection with satisfactory vaginal intercourse."[27]

Some clinical studies of male impotence actually delineate their definition of potency to include not only the ability to achieve an erection, but the frequency of this event and subsequent occurrence of a specific sexual activity. Similar to the other studies of heterosexist design, one team of researchers published their results in measuring the potency of men who had had their prostates surgically removed. "Patients were questioned preoperatively regarding the frequency of sexual intercourse with vaginal penetration. Even if a patient reported normal penile erections he was not considered to be sexually active if he was not engaging in vaginal intercourse."[28] By this disturbing definition, men who masturbate, have oral or anal sex, or engage in sex with men are not sexually active.

Another study invokes an unofficial scientific consensus that, "It is generally agreed . . . that vaginal penetration can be considered a suitable criterion of sexual potency."[29] This kind of medical focus on the desired goal of a successful erection or potency is quite limiting, given that both erotic sensation and orgasm can be achieved in the absence of an erection. This narrow scope of analysis devoted to the phallic insertive role mirrors much of the sexism in clinical trials involving heterosexual vaginal intercourse, where success is measured in terms of penile erection, vaginal penetration, and sometimes male ejaculation, but not clitoral stimulation or female orgasm.

Even though this article's analysis focuses on Viagra's impact on gay male cultures and sexual health, a variety of options have been available for treatment of erectile dysfunction in recent years. The medical studies mentioned previously attempt to assess several of these technologies, including the use of prosthetic implants, application of medication to the skin (transdermal), insertion of medication into the urethra, and injection of drugs directly into the erectile chambers of the penis.[30] The most popular form of injection therapy is marketed under the brand name Caverject. Delivered by injection, Caverject is inserted via syringe just beneath the skin at the base of the penis. Within a few minutes, the penis becomes erect regardless of physical or psychological stimulation (unlike Viagra) and can last more than an hour.

Caverject has been used for several years by gay men employed as sex workers. Although Viagra seems to have replaced Caverject on the set of porn video productions as the erectile drug of choice, Caverject remains popular due to its reliability, which is independent of erotic stimulation. Some men working as escorts in San Francisco and other cities obtain Caverject prescriptions and consider it a tool of the trade, ensuring an erection with any client at any time.

Representing yet another gap in the need for more comprehensive education on gay male sexual health, little attention has been given to the health concerns raised by Caverject. Some men use the drug more often than recommended out of economic necessity, risking tissue damage and other harmful consequences. The availability and cleanliness of syringes can be an issue when attempting to avoid sharing needles and potential blood-borne pathogens such as HIV. Breaking the skin of the penis at the base of the shaft (which may not be covered if a condom is used), just before sex, invites a heightened risk of sexually transmitted infection. Education targeting gay men who use Caverject without medical supervision would be a valuable component of public health outreach to these populations.

REAL MEN DON'T NEED VIAGRA

The use of Viagra also raises larger questions about the role of gender and masculinity in the quest for sexual potency. Technology now makes possible a pharmacological boost in one's manhood through the use of anabolic steroids, plastic surgery with pectoral and other implants to give the appearance of a muscular physique, and now the ability to control erections as never before. Gay men's appropriation of Viagra as a recreational drug used to enhance an already functioning sex drive and erectile capability, falls in line with a long tradition of hypermasculine social adaptation. Viagra raises the stakes in some men's quest for the ultimate masculinity, but already critiques of artificial manhood have begun to be voiced.

In what is surely the most extreme commentary on technologically aided masculinity to date, one physician calls for a return to "natural," power-wielding patriarchy rather than a reliance upon synthetic virility. David Saul is the director of the men's health program at the Midlife Health Centre in Toronto, and penned an opinion column titled "If Men Were Still Men, They Wouldn't Need Viagra" that was published in *The Toronto Star*. Critical of Viagra's popularity among aging men, he suggested that more natural means are readily available by maintaining an adequate level of testosterone production in the male body.

A decline in this production, he claims, can be prevented by engaging in four activities. These include: (1) muscle development, and not just from working out a gym. Apparently a gym physique is not a "real man" physique, for he prescribes musculature gained from work on a farm, in construction, or in the military—traditional bastions of tough guys. (2) One must also keep "sexually active," which he defines as every night. (3) "Maintain the position of decision-maker—head of the household, manager or supervisor at work, elder political statesman of the community." (4) "Maintain a hunter-gatherer type of nutrition."[31] (He goes on to list a manly dietary regimen.) In conclusion, Saul states that, "Men are not women. They don't look like women, act like women, think like women, or have sex like women. And they should not be forced into a woman's mold at the mid-life stage. Perhaps at 90, men can slow down and release the reins to the younger bucks. Until then, let men be the men that they were destined to be."[32]

With an adherence to a kind of gendered manifest destiny, Saul represents an extremist version of some popular culture values about sexual division of labor, the importance of virility in forging a link between masculinity and dominance, and the overall role of sexuality as a fundamental aspect of wielding power. In his world-view, resorting to Viagra use thwarts the masculine sustenance of necessary testosterone. Viagra is dangerous because it can indeed enable men who act like women (i.e., gay men) to have erections just like the men who do construction work, rule their community, keep the wife at home, and get laid nightly.

A common theme in the discourse surrounding Viagra has been exactly what Saul refers to when he speaks of ninety-year-old men and a reluctance to release their sexual reins to the "younger buck" generation. Although Saul's writing on this topic is presumably within a heterosexist context, a version of this issue exists for gay men as well. In the San Francisco community forum on Viagra use, Eric Rofes spoke of the countless gay male sexual spaces that have been established in previous decades and how many older gay men have abandoned communal sex in places like bathhouses, sex clubs, and more public sites due to erectile problems associated with age. Some of these men have left the sexual cultures they helped to create in the 1970s and 1980s, and Viagra may usher them back into their prior sexual activity. We may soon begin to see the implications for older gay men reentering sex scenes from which they have been commonly absent in the past.

While I have attempted to discern a number of the current and potential implications Viagra holds for gay men, pharmacology's impact on cultural practices is far from over as it relates to sexual potency. Many other erectile dysfunction treatments are in the development pipeline for eventual testing and FDA approval. Undoubtedly, as new health technologies in the forms of drugs and devices emerge, gay men's sexual health will continue to shift in unforeseen and perhaps dangerous directions unless an even closer relationship can be forged between gay community leaders and health science researchers.

SECTION IV:
CLEARING THE SMEAR

Immaculate Infection

So virginal like Mary,
it could only be Magic.
So guiltless in purity,
we are ever so tragic.

Our sweet cherubim faces
with Kaposi complexion,
such innocent victims of
immaculate infection.

We listened well to Nancy
when she chided, "Just Say No."
And you cared with such bias.
No one told us, "Told you so!"

We in positive sainthood
never tried drug injection,
we innocent victims of
immaculate infection.

Sacred Western blots confirm
like religious conversion.
Thank God we're married with kids,
clean and free from perversion.

Lord, how could this have happened?
Must be that bi connection.
How unfair to us straights with
immaculate infection.

Poor Kimberly Bergalis
wielded such justice Divine.
A true martyr made of Rock
compared to fairies who whine.

Forget dentist what's-his-name.
Please just mourn with selection
the elite privileged with
immaculate infection.

Only Whites (as in Ryan)
should warrant your attention,
not blacks and their green monkeys.
It was all their invention.

Ashe to ash and dust to dust,
we deserve resurrection
as innocent victims of
immaculate infection.

Chapter 6

Heterocopulative Syndrome: Clinico-Pathologic Correlation in 260 Cases

Michael Scarce

The following study, "Heterocopulative Syndrome: Clinico-Pathologic Correlation in 260 Cases," is reprinted from the fictional journal *Annals of Nuclear Family Clinical and Laboratory Science*, 6.1 (1998), pp. 1-6.[1]

ABSTRACT: The hazards of heterosexual behavior have been well documented. They include, but are not limited to, unplanned pregnancies, penile and cervical cancer, vaginitis, a host of sexually transmitted diseases (some of them incurable or deadly), a disproportionate propensity to engage in child molestation, global overpopulation, socially oppressive gender roles, and more. A recurring pattern of these health disorders resulting from the union of the penis and vagina has been named heterocopulative

---

1. The purpose of this parody is to articulate an oppositional narrative that reveals the laughable biases and social prejudice embedded in many medical science studies, often published as objective and unquestionable fact. Although this is an elementary strategy of turning the tables, it is nonetheless effective in demonstrating the continued prevalence of medical science's baseless assumptions, unfamiliarity with gay male cultures, and heterosexist methodology.

syndrome. These people could pose a serious public health threat if such practices continue unchecked and may be especially dangerous if employed as food handlers.[2]

PROBLEM AND LITERATURE REVIEW

Heterosexuals represent approximately 90 percent of the United States population, yet they account for well over 99 percent of the burdens faced by our health care system. Frequency, number, and dishonesty of sexual contacts among heterosexual men and women, which are facilitated at single's bars, church socials, and fraternity parties are cited by Stiffen and Stare as reasons for the emergence of new heterosexual diseases, as is their perception of heterosexuals as a "highly stagnant, immobile population" and " 'unnatural' sexual practices such as copulation, which allows transmission of a variety of organisms."[3] High rates of infidelity and a rising divorce rate in excess of 50 percent compound these risk factors.

For the sake of brevity, the term heterosexual practices will be used hereafter to denote penis-to-vagina copulation.[4] The fact that the patient has had or is now having homosexual relationships is irrelevant to the topic of discussion. Previous heterosexual activity,

---

2. The specter of the infectious food handler is frequently used as a medical basis for employment discrimination against gay, lesbian, bisexual, and transgendered people in the formulation of public policy and law. This form of discrimination against gay men is bolstered by the stereotype of the gay male employed as waiter or hospitality servant, representing a fear that gay men have infiltrated and now control every corner of the food service industry. Such fears also justify prominence in medical journal publication, for it purports to serve a larger social good.

3. Several medical publications attempt to use gay stereotypes to create epidemiological traffic patterns, citing the "well-known facts" that gay men travel and relocate residency more frequently, as well as their engagement in "bizarre" sexual practices such as fisting, rimming, and sadomasochism. Examples of this can be found in the work of Eric Z. Silfen and Thomas Stair, "Gay Bowel Syndrome: A Constellation of GI Disorders Peculiar to Homosexual Males," *Consultant*, July 1982, 85-94.

4. Many medical science publications use the term "homosexual practices" or "homosexuality" synonymously with penis-to-anus intercourse, as if this is the only (or even most popular) expression of same-sex sexual behavior. In addition, "homosexual" is often used in reference only to men, rendering lesbian women invisible or asexual.

even if represented by a single experience, exposes the patient to the conditions under consideration.[5]

METHOD

The subjects for this study were 260 heterosexual patients who visited a private family practice in a suburb of Salt Lake City, Utah, over the span of three years.[6] All of the patients were treated for some form of genitourinary affliction. Investigators reviewed the records of these patients, tabulating data on lab results, diagnoses, course of treatment, and demographic information. In addition, a survey instrument was designed to gain a sexual history from these heterosexuals. The form of the instrument was developed by modifying questions from our previous studies on homosexual health and cancer, and on the advice of one male heterosexual.[7] These forms of data collection were used to measure the multiple disorders and afflictions found with unusual frequency in male and female heterosexuals.

---

5. This is a parody of the classification provided by Norman Sohn and James Robilotti in "The Gay Bowel Syndrome: A Review of Colonic and Rectal Conditions in 200 Male Homosexuals," *American Journal of Gastroenterology* 675(5): 478-484 (1977). The fact that someone is currently engaging in heterosexual sex is deemed irrelevant by many researchers; a single same-sex experience in the patient's past is enough to taint the individual and permanently classify them as homosexual.

6. May studies conducted on gay men and infectious diseases use inner city, public, sexually transmitted disease clinics for their sample population. Too often these results are then generalized as a representation of all gay men regardless of socioeconomic status and geographic residence.

7. This is a parody of Janet Daling's study on homosexual practices and anal cancer, in which she attempts to establish the validity of her interview instrument by stating that it was developed by "modifying questions from our previous studies on *reproductive* health and cancer, from the questionnaire used by the San Francisco Sexually Transmitted Diseases Clinic, and *on the advice of a male homosexual*" (italics mine). It would be unthinkable for a peer-reviewed, medical science article to be published in a prestigious journal if the instrument used to measure heterosexual sex practices had been adapted from previous studies of nonreproductive health and based on the advice of a single heterosexual individual who is presumed to speak for all heterosexual people. See Janet Daling, Noel S. Weiss, T. Gregory Hislop, Christopher Maden, Ralph J. Coates, Karen J. Sherman, Rhoda L. Ashley, Marjorie Beagrie, John A. Ryan, and Lawrence Corey, "Sexual Practices, Sexually Transmitted Diseases, and the Incidence of Anal Cancer," *New England Journal of Medicine* 317(16): 973 (1987).

RESULTS

Clinical diagnoses of these patients included twenty conditions: vaginitis, yeast infections, impotence, delayed ejaculation, nongonococcal urethritis, abdominal cramping, unplanned or unwanted pregnancy, syphilis, urethral discharge, hepatitis B, irregular menstruation, delayed ejaculation, impotence, epididymitis, crab lice, chlamydia, human papillomavirus (HPV), HPV-related cancer, sterility, and physical trauma resulting from sexual assault.

DISCUSSION

There are certain physical findings which, while not absolutely diagnostic, should alert the examiner to the possibility of heterosexuality—pregnancy in women, diminished vaginal muscle tone, penile abrasions, expressed anxiety during prostate exams, female inability to achieve orgasm with her sexual partner, vasectomy, and more. An additional sign can be termed the Negative "O" Sign in which the male patient is incapable of voluntarily maintaining the anus in a dilated position. This sign was present in approximately 40 percent of the patients.[8]

Impotence was a common problem associated with heterocopulative syndrome in male heterosexuals. For the purposes of this study, impotence was defined as the lack of penile erection sufficient to engage in anal penetration.[9]

---

8. Again, see Sohn and Robilloti. They define the "O" sign as the ability to voluntarily maintain the anus in a dilated position, which in their research is a good indicator of the male patient's homosexuality.

9. Most clinical research on male erectile dysfunction defines potency as one study claims, "It is generally agreed . . . that vaginal penetration can be considered a suitable criterion of sexual potency," in Gunilla Ojdeby, Anders Claezon, Einar Brekkan, Michael Haggman, and Bo Johan Norlen, "Urinary Impotence and Sexual Impotence After Radical Prostatectomy," *Scandinavian Journal of Urology and Nephrology* 30: 473-477 (1966). This narrow scope of analysis devoted to the phallic insertive role mirrors much of the sexism in clinical trials involving heterosexual vaginal intercourse, where success is measured in terms of penile erection, vaginal penetration, and sometimes male ejaculation, but not clitoral stimulation or female orgasm.

In a study conducted by E. Stewart Geary, Theresa E. Dendinger, Fuad S. Freiha, and Thomas Stamey, "Nerve Sparing Radical Prostatectomy: A Different View," *Journal of Neurology* 154(1): 145-149 (July 1995), "Patients were questioned preoperatively regarding the frequency of sexual intercourse with vaginal penetration. Even if a patient reported normal penile erections he was not considered to be sexually active if he was not engaging in vaginal intercourse." By this disturbing definition, men who masturbate, have oral or anal sex, or engage in sex with men are not sexually active.

The typical patient has a history of multiple diseases accompanied by social dysfunction, which tend to recur. When alert to this clinical pattern, the physician may recognize the heterocopulative syndrome even before a history of heterosexuality has been elicited.

CONCLUSION

Physicians should broaden the scope of their medical examinations and diagnoses to encompass more than unplanned pregnancy, prostate cancer, and Pap smear screening when treating heterosexual patients. There is no doubt that our traditional conceptions of sexually transmitted diseases were too narrow; it is only slightly less certain that our current understanding of heterocopulative syndrome will expand and develop as new etiologies are implicated and new clinical syndromes described.[10] The public health implications of heterosexual behavior are very important. These patients may be employed as food handlers or in other roles where they could come into contact with others and spread a host of infectious and other conditions.

---

10. In the case of gay bowel syndrome, statements such as these reserve medical science's right to continuously update and revise the definitions of gay health and illness, while maintaining a space in which gay men can be perpetually objectified, fragmented, and scapegoated as responsible for any medical, and therefore social, problems which may arise. See Michael Heller, "The Gay Bowel Syndrome: A Common Problem of Homosexual Patients in the Emergency Department," *Annals of Emergency Medicine* 9(9): 492 (1980).

Chapter 7

Smear-Resistant Strategies

So how might we begin to clear these negligent, pathologizing, and disempowering smears that have been so damaging to the pleasure and health of queer sex? There persists a relative inability of activists to organize at the intersection of science and sexuality. While scholars in the fields of cultural studies, philosophy and history of science, and medical sociology, among others, have made great strides in laying the foundational work for holding health sciences more accountable, the subjugation of deviant sex is largely promoted by the gap between sociocultural theory and medical practice. This chasm presents a formidable obstacle with only scant and shakily built bridges of communication and collaboration.

The institutionalization of queer health provides one logical site for this work to take root. Great benefits could be reaped from a more sophisticated approach to sexual science through national professional organizations such as the Gay and Lesbian Medical Association, more grassroots and comprehensive health groups such as the National Lesbian and Gay Health Association, and the burgeoning reemergence of a strengthened network of gay and lesbian health clinics that hearken back to a late-1970s model of queer treatment, prevention, advocacy, and research advances literally housed under one roof.

Institutions also come with strings, however, and are usually accountable to some degree of popular opinion. When it comes to funding controversial research or harm reduction efforts, tapping privatized sources of individual donors and certain foundations may give some forms of advocacy a fighting chance. As the concept of a gay men's health movement continues to unfold, we must simultaneously conduct the necessary research to inform our organizing efforts. After all, the more we know about gay men's health, the better we can define our terms of progress. Research on these issues tends to be dismissed in academic settings, discouraged among health care professionals, outlawed throughout government agencies, and shamed from recognition as valid and valuable areas of inquiry.

The following outline represents an introductory, and by no means comprehensive, agenda to activism concerning science and gay men's sexual health, with an emphasis on broadening and integrating approaches to gay male wellness beyond the narrow scope of HIV and AIDS.

1. Critically examine biomedical claims that attribute AIDS and other disease susceptibility to biological origins of homosexuality.

While there is some utility in noting the specific health concerns amongst gay male populations that are higher in prevalence than national averages, we must retire the notion of gay diseases that are dependent upon some essential, physiological difference in gay men's bodies that, thus far, exists only in the scientific imagination. Coining an illness such as gay bowel syndrome might bring an individual researcher some amount of notoriety and journal publications, but the damage of branding an illness or collection of diseases as gay specific has wide-reaching implications far beyond the patient-provider relationship. Like it or not, health sciences are politically charged and highly influenced by nonscientific cultural forces. Likewise, the results of health science work are appropriated for political gains outside the laboratory or clinical setting.

Take, for example, the work of geneticist Dean Hamer who is best known for discovering the gay gene, even though no such discovery or determination has ever been made. Hamer's gay gene study was government funded through the National Cancer Research Institute under the guise of examining why gay men with AIDS seem to have higher rates of the skin cancer known as Kaposi's sarcoma as compared to the overall population of people with AIDS. His hypothesis rested on the suspicion that gay men must have a genetic makeup different from heterosexual men, thus contributing to a heightened susceptibility to certain forms of cancer. This suspected genetic factor was not portrayed in Hamer's published research findings as simply carcinogenic, however, but potentially causative of same-sex sexual orientation itself. Through the work of Hamer and others, desire and disease become inextricably linked as deviance is grounded in a constitutionally unhealthy body.

As scientists continue their search for the homosexual body through analyzing hormone levels, brain structures, fingerprints, inner ear structures, dental patterns, genetic makeup, and more, these hypothesized differences will undoubtedly continue to be attributed to the notion that gay men are somehow inherently diseased. Mounting an opposition that analyzes and critiques homophobic science, which is increasingly conducted by scientists who are gay themselves, almost seems an insurmountable feat at times. The privileging of medical authority in the United States over the last hundred years has catapulted biomedical scientists to a level synonymous with religious leaders. They define our world, explain it, unraveling it before our eyes. Any opposition or claims to the contrary that originate from outside a strict and formulaic peer review constitutes nothing short of heresy. The very definition of gay and the meaning of gay men's health is at stake as scientific knowledge continues to be constructed in such a way that tells a particular kind of story about where gay men come from and what forces ultimately determine their existence.

2. Demand aggressive research, development, and approval of new and prospective sexual technologies.

A brief look at the recent history of AIDS has taught us a valuable lesson: public health work must not exclusively focus on behavioral mechanisms for prevention. Rather than simply encourage people to make different sexual choices for the betterment of their health, we should also begin to develop new technologies that enable people to engage in the same behaviors more safely or expand their menu of available options. Devices such as internal condoms and substances such as rectal microbicides provide two excellent examples of technology's potential to revolutionize sexual behavior.

The enablement of safer sex should not be the only goal, however. Technologies that have no impact on the health of sexual behavior, but enable or enhance the pleasure of that behavior, should also be prioritized. The popular slogan "Be here for the cure" epitomizes how the value of sexuality is erased or dismissed. Within the domain of AIDS rhetoric, the goal of a cure or vaccine is invariably framed only in a context of survival. Extending the lives of gay men is a crucial pursuit, but not once have I read or heard a single AIDS expert envisioning a future in which HIV and other sexually transmitted infections are so preventable and conquerable that gay men could return to fucking without condoms. Not once have we allowed ourselves to publicly wish for unprotected sex without health consequences, let alone set our sights on achieving that long-term, illustrious goal.

3. Demand better biomedical research on the sexual transmission of disease.

We still do not have a clear understanding of the presence, risk, or viral load of HIV in pre-seminal fluid. Almost twenty years into the epidemic, no one can begin to estimate the role of pre-cum in seroconversion. Parallel uncertainties continue with respect to vaginal fluid and menstrual blood. No one knows if rectal douching before or after anal sex might reduce or exacerbate the risk of sexually transmitted infection. Gay men have been asking relatively simple and basic questions for at least twenty years about their sexual health in an attempt to make informed decisions about the management of risk and safety with their sex. Most of this area of inquiry remains uncharted, and not because of any scientific impossibility of generating answers.

Research dollars from private sources should become a new priority, for gay men can no longer sit back and hope for unlikely government or university approval of monies to research and enable healthier "criminal activity" (i.e., sodomy). The role of human papilloma virus in the etiology of anorectal cancer in gay men who practice receptive anal intercourse, the sexual transmission and natural history of Hepatitis C, the risk and process of HIV infection via the urethra in HIV-negative tops who penetrate HIV-negative bottoms, and more elaborate research on the mouth and pharynx as sites of HIV exposure are just a few of the unknowns that demand more complex and extensive knowledge.

4. Broaden the public health scope of gay male health and wellness beyond AIDS.

For too long, gay male health has been viewed solely through the limiting lens of HIV infection. The outpouring of research dollars and other funding for AIDS has yielded some of the most important data collection and scholarship ever conducted on gay men's lives. The relationship between gay men and the health sciences has never been more intimate. The limitations of this work, however, have included a narrow focus on gay male health and sexuality only as it relates to HIV infection. New treatments that prolong the lives of many HIV-positive gay men have had a profound and disorienting effect on the health sciences. While clearly a sign of progress, the latest drug regimens seem to have complicated treatment, prevention, and research work in unprecedented and unforeseen ways. At the same time, a lull in sickness and death rates has allowed gay communities to collectively catch their breath and turn their attention to other pressing health concerns that have been neglected in the wake of AIDS.

Certainly work on issues related to antigay violence, substance abuse, sexually transmitted infections, mental health, and other concerns has continued during the last two decades of AIDS, but almost never in a well-connected and integrated network. Few cities and even fewer states have organized gay health task forces or any kind of structured collaboration around the health issues faced by gay men's communities. Although there are national professional associations for gay health workers, there is no national scientific research agenda on gay men's health, let alone a queer equivalent of Healthy People 2000. In fact, the Healthy People 2010 document mentions gay men only twice—and only in relation to AIDS. Lesbians, bisexuals, and transgender people are not mentioned at all.

Where is the national campaign to educate and encourage gay men to get vaccinated for Hepatitis A and B? Where are the community clinics' free screenings for parasites? Where is the outreach to gyms with a largely gay clientele to do prevention and harm reduction work on steroid abuse and body image issues? Furthermore, why limit health work targeting gay men to sexually specific concerns? Why don't we see more health organizations doing outreach to gay men, offering low-cost services such as free flu shots, cholesterol checks, or tobacco cessation education? Why is it nearly impossible to find a self-defense course for gay men in most urban areas? Constructing a public health response to the needs of gay men must move beyond handing out condoms in bars and offering HIV-antibody testing at gay pride events.

5. Gay men must become engaged allies with women's health movements, and not just with lesbian health issues.

The Reality Female Condom, anal Pap smears, and internal microbicides are just a few examples which demonstrate just how closely intertwined the health of women and gay men have become within the overlapping realms of science and sexuality. Gay men have always stood to learn a great deal from feminist health movements and feminist approaches to science and technology. The scientific subordination of gay men's sexualized bodies under the medical gaze need not be tackled in a vacuum, and a toolbox of sorts already exists for organizing opposition to heterosexism and homophobia in health science methodology, protocol, and pedagogy. Beyond simply borrowing from feminism, gay men also have a great deal to contribute to women's health movements in the forms of resources, moral support, and political alliance.

6. Continue to investigate and democratize health sciences research, policy, and practice, as well as the management of their sociocultural implications.

Why has the United States Food and Drug Administration never approved a single safer sex device—including the latex condom—for anal sex? How is it that health science researchers can get away with defining a "successful erection" as the ability to penetrate a vagina? Why do pharmaceutical companies need FDA approval to use slang language that is culturally competent and accessible to gay male communities in educating physicians about lethal drug interactions? How can a gay man with colon cancer be misdiagnosed as having gay bowel syndrome simply because of his sexual orientation? Why have there been two illnesses with official gay names (GBS and GRID), while there has never been an illness with a heterosexual-specific nomenclature? Why is the pursuit of internal microbicides for STD prophylaxis being restrictively labeled as female controlled safer sex technology, as if men are never penetrated sexually? Why are gay men denied official, sanctioned access to new safer sex technologies on a national level based on antiquated sodomy laws in some states?

In many ways, the crisis years of AIDS have positioned gay men's lives squarely in the domain of the health sciences. The increasing influence of technology on our lives, a health care system suffering a crisis of its own, and the expanding cultural authority of science should all serve as a clarion call for greater involvement in the problematic relationship between gay male sexuality and the health sciences. Sexual health underpins gay men's individual and collective ability to thrive. We must never underestimate or fail to defend how the pleasure we give each other fortifies that pursuit to no end.

Notes

Introduction

1. Anne Fausto-Sterling. *Myths of Gender: Biological Theories About Women and Men* (New York: BasicBooks, 1992), 224.

2. See Eric Rofes. *Dry Bones Breathe: Gay Men Creating Post-AIDS Identities and Cultures* (Binghamton, NY: The Haworth Press, Inc., 1998).

Chapter 1

1. See also: Ludwick Fleck. *Genesis and Development of a Scientific Fact* (Chicago: University of Chicago Press, 1979); and Bruno Latour. *Science in Action: How to Follow Scientists and Engineers Through Society* (Cambridge, MA: Harvard University Press, 1987).

2. Jennifer Terry and Jacqueline Urla. "Introduction: Mapping Embodied Deviance." In Jennifer Terry and Jacqueline Urla (Eds.), *Deviant Bodies: Critical Perspectives on Difference in Science and Popular Culture* (Bloomington, IN: Indiana University Press, 1995), 1.

3. While I use the singularity of "a subculture" here, I do not seek to negate the diversity of gay urban cultural groupings of the 1970s around class, race, ethnicity, fetishisms, sexual practices, and more. The medical uses of language of homogenization in reference to urban gay men furthers my argument in bringing to light the ways in which gay men are lumped together as a classification of bodies, behaviors, identities, and diseases without regard to individual or intracultural differences and affinities.

4. Steven Epstein. "Moral Contagion and the Medicalizing of Gay Identity: AIDS in Historical Perspective," *Research in Law, Deviance, and Social Control* 9: 1-42 (1987).

5. Paula Treichler. "AIDS, Homophobia, and Biomedical Discourse: An Epidemic of Signification." In Douglas Crimp (Ed.), *AIDS: Cultural Analysis, Cultural Activism* (Cambridge, MA: MIT Press, 1988), 37.

6. This debut was not without a series of preceding dress rehearsals, however. See H. Most. "Manhattan: A Tropical Isle?" *The American Journal of Tropical Medicine and Hygiene* 17(3): 333-354 (1968).

7. Henry L. Kazal, Norman Sohn, Jose I. Carrasco, James G. Robilotti, and William E. Delaney. "The Gay Bowel Syndrome: Clinico-Pathologic Correlation in 260 Cases," *Annals of Clinical and Laboratory Science* 6(2): 185 (1976).

8. *Ibid.,* 189.

9. Norman Sohn and James G. Robilotti. "The Gay Bowel Syndrome: A Review of Colonic and Rectal Conditions in 200 Male Homosexuals," *American Journal of Gastroenterology* 67(5): 478 (1977). Reprinted with permission from the American College of Gastroenterology. *American Journal of Gastroenterology,* (1977.)

10. *Ibid.*

11. Michael Heller. "The Gay Bowel Syndrome: A Common Problem of Homosexual Patients in the Emergency Department," *Annals of Emergency Medicine* 9(9): 492 (1980).

12. See P.O. Pehrson and A. Bjorkman. "The 'Gay Bowel Syndrome' and Amebiasis as Sexually Transmitted Diseases in Sweden," *Lakartidningen* 78(35): 2924 (1981); John C. Kaufman and Sidney M. Fierst. "Shigellosis and the Gay Bowel Syndrome: An Endoscopic Point of View and Review of the Literature," *Gatrointestinal Endoscopy* 28(4): 250-251 (1982); Eric Z. Silfen and Thomas Stair. "Gay Bowel Syndrome: A Constellation of GI Disorders Peculiar to Homosexual Males," *Consultant,* July 1982(7), 85-94; Alan H. Friedman, Juan Orellana, William R. Freeman, Maurice H. Luntz, Michael B. Starr, Michael L. Tapper, Ilya Sigland, Heidrum Rotterdam, Ricardo Mesa Tejada, Susan Braunhut, et al. "Cytomegalovirus Retinitis: A Manifestation of the Acquired Immune Deficiency Syndrome (AIDS)," *British Journal of Ophthalmology* 67(6): 372-380 (1983); Thomas C. Quinn. "Gay Bowel Syndrome: The Broadened Spectrum of Nongenital Infection," *Postgraduate Medicine* 76(2): 197-210 (August 1984); Wilmer Rodriguez. "Gay Bowel Syndrome," *Boletin—Associacion Medica de Puerto Rico* 78(10): 439-441 (October, 1986); Barbara E. Laughon, Dolph A. Druckman, Andrew Vernon, Thomas C. Quinn, B. Frank Polk, John F. Modlin, Robert H. Yolken, and John G. Bartlett. "Prevalence of Enteric Pathogens in Homosexual Men With and Without Acquired Immunodeficiency Syndrome," *Gastroenterology* 94(4): 984-993 (1988); Bruce S. Gingold. "Gay Bowel Syndrome: An Overview." In Pearl Ma and Donald Armstrong (Eds.), *AIDS and Infections of Homosexual Men* (Stoneham, MA: Butterworth, 1989), 49-58; J.Y. Kang, D. Stiel, and W.F. Doe. "Proctolitis Caused by Concurrent Amoebiasis and Gonococcal Infection: The 'Gay Bowel Syndrome,'" *The Medical Journal of Australia* 2(9): 496-497 (1979); and P. Paulet and G. Stoffels. "Maladies anorectales sexuellement transmissibles, [Sexually-transmissable anorectal diseases]," *Review Medicale de Bruxelles,* 10(8): 327-334 (1989).

13. Heller, *op. cit.,* p. 487.

14. Kazal et al., *op. cit.,* p. 192.

15. Sohn and Robilotti, *op. cit.,* p. 478.

16. D. E. Whitley. *STDs: Sexually Transmitted Diseases* (Arlington, TX: Fairview Publications, 1993), 42.

17. J.H. Caldwell. (1985). "The Gay Bowel Syndrome." In V. A. Spagna and R. B. Prior (Eds.), *Sexually Transmitted Diseases: A Clinical Syndrome Approach* (New York: Marcel Dekker), 256.

18. Cindy Patton. *Inventing AIDS* (New York: Routledge, 1990), 119.

19. Gay historian Jonathan Ned Katz offers a comprehensive analysis of the initial deviance and subsequent normalizing of heterosexuality as an identity and a practice in *The Invention of Heterosexuality* (New York: Dutton, 1995).

20. Simon Watney. "The Spectacle of AIDS." In Douglas Crimp (Ed.), *AIDS: Cultural Analysis, Cultural Activism* (Cambridge, MA: MIT Press), 79.

21. Silfen and Stair, *op. cit.,* p. 86.

22. Yu Men Chen, Michael Davis, and David J. Ott. "Traumatic Rectal Hematoma Following Anal Rape," *Annals of Emergency Medicine* 15(7): 850-852 (July 1986).

23. For more on the conflation between adult male rape and consensual homo sex, see Michael Scarce. *Male on Male Rape: The Hidden Toll of Stigma and Shame* (New York: Plenum); and Richie McMullen. *Male Rape: Breaking the Silence on the Last Taboo* (Boston: Alyson Publications, 1990).

24. Jennifer Terry. "Anxious Slippages Between 'Us' and 'Them': A Brief History of the Scientific Search for Homosexual Bodies." In Jennifer Terry and Jacqueline Urla (Eds.), *Deviant Bodies* (Bloomington, IN: Indiana University Press, 1995), 129.

25. Kazal et al., *op. cit.,* p. 191.

26. For more on the vulnerable rectum/fragile urethra/rugged vagina paradigm, see John Langone. "AIDS," *Discover* 6(12): 28-53 (December 1985); and Paula Treichler's critical analysis of this concept in "AIDS, Homophobia, and Biomedical Discourse: An Epidemic of Signification." In Douglas Crimp (Ed.). *AIDS: Cultural Analysis, Cultural Activism* (Cambridge, MA: MIT Press); and Michael Fumento. *The Myth of Heterosexual AIDS* (New York: Basic Books, 1990).

27. Leo Bersani. "Is the Rectum a Grave?" In Douglas Crimp (Ed.). *AIDS: Cultural Analysis, Cultural Activism* (Cambridge, MA: MIT Press); and Michael Fumento. *The Myth of Heterosexual AIDS* (New York: Basic Books, 1990), 211.

28. Randy Shilts, "A New Plague on Our House: Gastro-Intestinal Diseases," *The Advocate*, April 20, 1977, p. 12.

29. C.L. Thomas (Ed.). *Taber's Cyclopedic Medical Dictionary,* Sixteenth Edition (Philadelphia: F. A. Davis Company, 1989), 1804.

30. Kang, et al.

31. Jan Zita Grover. "AIDS: Keywords." In Douglas Crimp (Ed.). *AIDS: Cultural Analysis, Cultural Activism* (Cambridge, MA: MIT Press), 19.

32. Heller, *op. cit.,* p. 492.

33. Quinn, *op. cit.*; Silfen and Stair, *op. cit.*; and Friedman, *op. cit.*

34. Sohn and Robilotti, *op. cit.,* p. 482.

35. *Ibid.*

36. Kazal et al., *op. cit.,* p. 185.

37. Thomas, *op. cit.,* p. 1804.

38. Silfen and Stair, *op. cit.,* pp. 85-86.

39. Kazal et al., *op. cit.,* p. 185.

40. Sohn and Robilotti, *op. cit.,* p. 483.

41. Heller, *op. cit.,* p. 487.

42. Robin Marantz Henig. "AIDS: A New Disease's Deadly Odyssey," *The New York Times*, February 6, 1983, Sec. 6, p. 28.

43. Dennis L. Breo. "Confronting AIDS: Blunt Facts About an Insidious Killer and What You Need to Know to Protect Yourself," *Chicago Tribune*, April 26, 1987, C14.

44. Shilts 1977, *op. cit.,* p. 12.

45. John Crewdson. "Weak Immune System May Open AIDS Door," *Chicago Tribune*, December 20, 1987, C1.

46. Andy Dabilis. "The Guys Are Scared Silly . . . They're Dying," United Press International, August 9, 1982.

47. *Ibid.*

48. See also Donna Haraway's writings on cross-species transgressions, identification, and relations with nonhuman others in *Primate Visions: Gender, Race, and Nature in the World of Modern Science* (New York: Routledge, 1989).

49. Patton, *op. cit.,* p. 28.

50. Randy Shilts. *And the Band Played On* (New York: St. Martin's Press, 1987), 71.

51. "Opportunistic Diseases: A Puzzling New Syndrome Afflicts Homosexual Men," *Time*, December 21, 1981, p. 68.

52. Michael S. Gottlieb, Robert Schroff, Suzanna Fligiel, John L. Fahey, and Andrew Saxon. "Gay-Related Immunodeficiency (GRID) Syndrome: Clinical and Autopsy Observations," *Clinical Research* 30(2): 349A (1982).

53. Lawrence Mass. "Some Good News: VD Rates Are Down," *New York Native*, April 11, 1983, p. 19.

54. Bobby Campbell. "Gay Lymph-Node Syndrome," *San Francisco Sentinel*, May 13, 1982, p. 6.

55. G. Barbedette. "French notes on AIDS," *New York Native*, June 4, 1983, p. 24.

56. Campbell, p. 6.

57. R.O. Brennan and D.T. Durack. "Gay Compromise Syndrome," *Lancet*, 2(8259) (1981): 1338-1339.

58. For a more thorough discussion of essentialism, gay and lesbian identity, and disease, see Stephen Epstein. "Nature vs. Nurture and the Politics of AIDS Organizing," *Out/Look* 1(3): 46-53 (1988). In this article, Epstein also elaborates the ways in which the shared experience of AIDS has further increased the ethnic identification of gay communities. He suggests maintaining a creative tension between essentialism and constructionism, using the contradictions as a valuable strategy in the struggle against AIDS.

59. Pamela Murphy. Regional News. United Press International, April 15, 1982.

60. James E. D'Eramo. "Treating the Syndrome, Not the Infection," *New York Native,* August 1, 1983, p. 22.

61. Richard B. Pearce. "Parasites and AIDS," *New York Native*, August 29, 1983, p. 26. Italics mine.

62. Tom Bethell. "Rethinking HIV," *American Spectator*, June 1993, p. 13.

63. Laughon et al., *op. cit.*

64. See John Greyson's film *Zero Patience* for a critical exploration of the historical construction of Gaetan Dugas into the character of Patient Zero.

65. Wlliam W. Darrow. "In Memoriam," *Journal of Sex Research* 31(3): 248 (1994).

66. Larry Kramer's late 1970s novel *Faggots* (New York: Plume, 1978) about gay sexual decadence in New York City is often characterized in hindsight by AIDS writers and critics as a prophecy of impending self-destruction. Kramer does not simply imply disease as as catastrophic consequence, he uses it as a narrative tool to foreshadow the supposed breakdown of civilized gay life.

67. Robert Knight. Testimony presented to the United States Committee on Labor and Human Resources by Robert H. Knight, Director, Cultural Studies the Family Research Council, *Federal Document Clearing House Congressional Testimony*, July 29, 1994.

68. Dabilis, *op. cit.*

69. Grover, *op. cit.,* p. 23.

70. Pat Buchanan. "Hunting Cures," *Time*, July 25, 1983, p. 4.

71. Karen Jo Gounaud. "The Real Meaning of the Word 'Anti-Gay,'" *The Washington Times,* March 23, 1994, p. C2.

72. Michael Sharman. "The Homosexual Lifestyle is a Dangerous One," *National Law Journal*, Feburary 27, 1995, p. A20.

73. William E. Dannemeyer. "Gays in the Military," *Chicago Tribune*, December 23, 1991, p. C21.

74. William E. Dannemeyer. *Shadow In the Land* (San Francisco: Ignatius Press, 1989), 219.

75. Paul Cameron. *Medical Consequences of What Homosexuals Do* (Pamphlet published by the Family Research Insititute, Washington, DC, 1993).

76. Trevor Lautens. "The 'Love' We Dare Not Defame," *Vancouver Sun*, April 8, 1983, p. A21.

77. Samuel P. Woodward. "Adoption Not Intended to Help Homosexuals' Self-Esteem," *The Columbian*, July 5, 1995, p. A11. Italics mine.

78. Whitley, *op. cit.,* p. 42.

79. Mass, *op. cit.,* p. 19.

80. Rick O'Keefe, Peter Marcus, Janet Townsend, and Marji Gold. "Use of the Term 'Gay Bowel Syndrome,'" *American Family Physician* 49(3): 580 (1983).

81. Glen E. Hastings and Richard Weber. "In Reply to 'Use of the Term Gay Bowel Syndrome' Letter," *American Family Physician* 49(3): 582 (1993). Italics mine.

82. *Ibid.*

83. Grover, *op. cit.,* p. 28.

84. Kang, Stiel, Doe, *op. cit.,* pp. 496-497.

85. Pehrson and Bjorkman, *op. cit.,* p. 2924.

86. L. Prufer-Kramer and A. Kramer. "Gastrointestinale Manifestationen von AIDS. Teil 1: Grundlagen und Virale Infektionen. [Gastrointestinal manifesta-

tions of AIDS 1: Basic considerations and viral infections,]" *Fortschritte der Medizin* 109(7): 169-172 (1991).

87. Friedman et al., *op. cit.*

88. Paulet and Stoffels, *op. cit.*

89. Rodriguez, *op. cit.*

90. See also Simon Watney's essay on "Re-Gaying AIDS" in his book *Practices of Freedom: Selected Writings on HIV/AIDS* (Durham, NC: Duke University Press, 1994); as well as Edward King's *Safety in Numbers: Safer Sex and Gay Men* (New York: Routledge, 1993) and Eric Rofes's *Reviving the Tribe: Regenerating Gay Men's Sexuality and Culture in the Ongoing Epidemic* (Binghamton, NY: The Haworth Press, Inc., 1996). See also Eric Rofes. "Gay Lib vs. AIDS: Averting Civil War in the 1990s" in Mark Blasius and Shane Phelan (Eds.) (1997). *We Are Everywhere: A Historical Sourcebook of Gay and Lesbian Politics* (New York: Routledge), 652-659.

91. Gregg Bordowtiz has written on the differences between confession and testimony, as well as the construction of identity through disease. See his article "Dense Moments" in Rodney Sappington and Tyler Stallings (Eds.). *Uncontrollable Bodies: Testimonies of Identity and Culture* (Seattle, WA: Bay Press, 1994), 25-44.

Chapter 2

1. Judith Butler. *Bodies That Matter: On the Discursive Limits of "Sex"* (New York: Routledge, 1993), 239.

2. *Ibid.*

3. Paul Raeburn. "Female Condom—FDA," Associated Press, December 13, 1993.

4. Robert G. Jobst and Judith S. Johns. "Investigation of an Inserted Anal Condom (Aegis) for the Receptive Partner Involved in Anal Sex," (unpublished report from a research study conducted at Howard Brown Memorial Health Clinic of Chicago, 1991), 2224.

5. *Ibid.,* 2230.

6. *Ibid.,* 2227.

7. David Tuller. "Health Department to Distribute Gay Condom," *San Francsisco Chronicle,* April 1, 1996, p. A13.

8. *Ibid.,* A14.

9. C. Davidson. "Does Reality Bite?" *POZ*, October/November, 1994, p. 55.

10. W. Buchignani, "A condom for her? Naturally, we're curious . . ." *The Montreal Gazette*, January 26, 1992, p. A1.

11. Edward King. *Safety in Numbers: Safer Sex and Gay Men* (London: Routledge, 1990), 98.

12. Jane Meredith Adams. "On Conference Fringe, Condoms for Women, Cases of Frustration," *The Boston Globe*, June 25, 1990, p. A8. Italics mine.

13. Beth Coleman. "Packaging Reality: Is the Female Condom Better Than We've Been Told?" *Village Voice,* May 19, 1993, p. 25.

14. Wisconsin Pharmacal Press Release. Chicago, IL.

15. "Female Condom Approved," *FDA Bulletin* (Department of Health and Human Services: Food and Drug Administration), June 22, 1993.

16. Food and Drug Administration, "Statement by the Food and Drug Administration," United States Department of Health and Human Services, April 27, 1993.

17. "Aegis Barrier Pouch: Instructions for Use." Booklet produced by Wisconsin Pharmacal Company for research conducted in 1992 at Howard Brown Memorial Clinic in Chicago, Illinois.

18. Cindy Patton. *Inventing AIDS* (London: Routledge, 1990), 188.

19. Text quoted from the Web site of "Joe," titled *Bearhunt*, which can be found on the World Wide Web at: http://www.xs4all.nl/~joe/bear/bear3/sexual. htm. For an opposing review, see Dan Savage's advice column, "Savage Love," *Village Voice*, August 12, 1997, p. 107.

20. "Condoms for Bottoms," *International Drummer* 196: 52 (1996). See also Jayson Marston. "Bagged by Reality: How Good Are Vaginal Condoms for Ass Fucking?" *International Drummer* 205: 13 (1997).

21. *Bearhunt, op. cit.*

22. Sarah Strickland. "Gay Men Turn to the Female Contraceptive," *The Observer*, December 12, 1993, p. 13.

23. "Condoms for Bottoms."

24. *Bearhunt, op. cit.*

25. *Bearhunt, op. cit.*

26. "Female Condom Gains Favor Among Gays, But Effectiveness Unproven," (New York: Associated Press), June 26, 1996.

27. Charles Silverstein and Edmund White. *The Joy of Gay Sex* (New York: Crown, 1977), 143.

28. R.D. Fenwick. *Advocate Guide to Gay Health* (Boston: Alyson, 1982), 67.

29. G. Hannon, "A Bum Wrap," *Xtra!*, December 6, 1991, p. 3. For a more detailed analysis of the survey's results, see Steven Gibson, William McFarland, Dan Wohlfeiler, Kurt Scheer, and Mitchell H. Katz. (1999). "Experiences of 100 Men Who Have Sex with Men Using the Reality Condom for Anal Sex," *AIDS Education and Prevention* 11(1): 65-71.

30. Suzanne Sataline. "A Lonely Few Roam the Night to Save Lives," *Philadelphia Inquirer*, September 22, 1995, p. A1.

31. Stephen Gibson. "Anal Condom Survey—Preliminary Results," Stop AIDS Project unpublished document, August 2, 1997.

32. Cynthia Laird. "Getting a Reality Check: Anal Condoms Rank High Among Gay Men," *Bay Area Reporter*, August 7, 1997, p. 1.

33. Gibson, *op. cit.*

34. Michael Gross, S.P. Buchbinder, S. Holte, C. Celum, and B.A. Koblin. (1998). "Use of Reality Condoms for Anal Sex by HIV-Seronegative US Gay/ Bisexual Men at Increased Risk of HIV Infection," poster presentation given at 12th World AIDS Conference in Geneva, Switzerland. Abstract number 33128.

35. Douglas T. Newberry. "Femidoms and Gay Men," *Straight Talk: The Newsletter of Salisbury Gay Men's Health Project* 4:7, 1996.

36. Mitch Katz, March 19, 1996. Memorandum from Director of Epidemiology, Disease Control and AIDS of the City and County of San Francisco's Department of Public Health AIDS Office.

37. Instructional flyer produced by the San Francisco Department of Health distributed in San Francisco, 1996.

38. Gabriel Rotello. "Our Little Secret," *The Advocate*, April 16, 1996, p. 72.

39. For those wishing to explore this method of payment, the MediCal billing code is X6; the product code is 9914P; and the manufacturer code 11423X6.

40. Personal interview with Marcy Fraser conducted in San Francisco on November 20, 1996.

41. "Gays Using Anal Condoms," Associated Press, June 25, 1996.

42. Sarah Strickland. "Gay Men Turn to the Female Contraceptive," *The London Observer*, December 12, 1993, p. 13.

43. This definition of magpie is quoted from *Random House Compact Unabridged Dictionary,* Second Edition.

44. Strickland, *op. cit.,* p. 13.

45. Lisa M. Krieger. "Men Offered Condom Made for Women: S.F. Clinics Giving Devices to Gays Though They're Not OK'd for Male Use," *The San Francisco Examiner*, March 7, 1996, p. A3.

46. *Ibid.*

47. Mike Salinas. "Female Condoms for Male-Male Sex: FDA Denies Reality to Gays," *Bay Area Reporter,* February 29, 1996, pp. 1 and 26.

48. Robin Gorna. *Vamps, Virgins, and Victims: How Can Women Fight AIDS?* (London: Cassell, 1995), 390.

49. Mitch Katz, March 19, 1996. Memorandum from Director of Epidemiology, Disease Control and AIDS of the City and County of San Francisco's Department of Public Health AIDS Office.

50. Mike Salinas. "Internal Condoms Available Now: San Francisco Men Get Some Reality," *Bay Area Reporter*, March 7, 1996, p. 15.

51. Paul Raeburn. "Female Condom—FDA," Associated Press, December 13, 1993.

52. *Ibid.*

53. Salinas, *op. cit.,* p. 15.

54. *Op. cit.*

55. Gorna, *op. cit.,* 1997, p. 298.

56. Beth Silverman and Thomas Gross. "Use and Effectiveness of Condoms During Anal Intercourse: A Review," *Sexually Transmitted Diseases* 24(1): 15 (1997).

Chapter 3

1. J. Kreiss, E. Ngugi, K. Holmes, J. Ndinya-Achola, P. Waiyaki, P.L. Roberts, I. Ruminjo, R. Sajabi, J. Kimata, T.R. Fleming, et al. "Efficacy of N-9 Con-

traceptive Sponge Use in Preventing Heterosexual Acquisition of HIV in Nairobi Prostitutes," *Journal of American Medical Association* 268(4): 477-482 (1992).

2. Anastasia Stephens. "Gel That Gives Peace of Mind," *Daily Mall* (London), October 21, 1997, p. 40.

3. Department of Health and Human Services Press Release, "Shalala Announces HIV Prevention Initiative; Calls for Accelerated Effort on Microbicides," July 9, 1996. For more on the call for microbicide development, see C.J. Elias and L.L. Heise. "Challenges for the Development of Female-Controlled Vaginal Microbicides," *AIDS 1994* 9(1): 1-9 (1994); Malcolm Potts. "The Urgent Need for a Vaginal Microbicide in the Prevention of HIV Transmission," *American Journal of Public Health* 84(6): 890-891 (1994); and David C. Sokal and Paul L. Hermonat. "Priorities for Vaginal Microbicide Research," *American Journal of Public Health* 85(5): 737-738 (1995).

4. Richard A. Knox. "AIDS Scientists Pin Hopes on Topical Agent; U.S. Pledges $100m Toward Development of Preventive Measure for Women," *The Boston Globe*, July 10, 1996, p. 4. Reprinted courtesy of *The Boston Globe*. While this essay focuses on anal sex practiced by gay men, the possible benefits of rectal microbicides for heterosexual anal sex are valuable and noteworthy as well, especially in other countries where the predominant mode of HIV transmission is heterosexual intercourse.

5. Cindy Patton. *Fatal Advice: How Safe-Sex Education Went Wrong* (Durham, NC: Duke University Press, 1996), 97.

6. See G. Hart et al. "Relapse to Unsafe Sexual Behaviour Among Gay Men: A Critique of Recent Behavioural HIV/AIDS Research," *Sociology of Health and Illness* 14(2): 216-232 (1992); Walt Odets. "Why We Stopped Doing Primary Prevention for Gay Men in 1985," *AIDS and Public Policy Journal* 9(1): 1-18 (1995); and Jack Morin. *Anal Pleasure and Health: A Guide for Men and Women*, Third Edition (San Francisco: Down There Press, 1998); and Eric Rofes's speech titled "The Emerging Sex Panic Targeting Gay Men," delivered at the National Gay and Lesbian Task Force's Creating Change Conference in San Diego, California, on November 16, 1997.

7. Michelangelo Signorile. "Bareback and Reckless," *OUT*, July 1997, p. 39. Similarly hysterical journalism on barebacking includes Marc Peyser, Elizabeth Roberts, and Frappa Stout, "A Deadly Dance," *Newsweek*, September 29, 1997, p. 76; Mubarak Dahir, "Sometimes Words Really Can Hurt You," *The Philadelphia Gay News*, January 13, 1998, p. 6; Dan Perreten, "The Bareback Phenomenon," *Windy City Times*, May 29, 1997, p. 3.

8. Eric Rofes. *Dry Bones Breathe: Gay Men Creating Post-AIDS Identities and Cultures* (Binghamton, NY: The Haworth Press, Inc., 1998), 148.

9. Kate Shindle. "Barebacking? Brainless," *The Advocate*, February 3, 1998, p. 9. Italics mine.

10. James W. Dilley, William J. Woods, and William McFarland. "Are Advances in Treatment Changing Views About High-Risk Sex?" *New England Journal of Medicine* 337(7): 501-502 (1997).

11. In late 1997, Kate Shindle was quoted as saying, "I don't endorse needle exchanges because they really sort of break the law. I do support teaching people how to clean needles and educating people on how to start protecting themselves. But as far as giving needles to the public, I'm not in support of that" (*The Washington Post*, September 14, 1997). To her credit, Shindle later reversed her stance and became a strong advocate for both condom distribution and needle exchange programs.

12. Rofes traces this evolution in his book *Reviving the Tribe: Regenerating Gay Men's Sexuality and Culture in the Ongoing Epidemic* (Binghamton, NY: The Haworth Press, Inc., 1995).

13. Knox, *op. cit.,* p. 4.

14. Jennifer Kornreich. "Iffy Lube," *Village Voice,* April 14, 1998, p. 53.

15. *Ibid.*

16. Richard Locke. "Riding Bareback," *PWA Coalition Newsline* (Fort Lauderdale), November 1997, pp. 7 and 11.

17. Clark L. Taylor. "Bringing Safe Sex Up to Date," *Bay Area Reporter,* May 22, 1997, p. 6.

18. Robin Gorna. *Vamps, Virgins, and Victims: How Can Women Fight AIDS?* (London: Cassell, 1995), 307.

19. Clark Taylor. (1998). "HIV/STD Prevention, Topical microbicides and Rectal Sex," poster presentation given at 12th World AIDS Conference in Geneva, Switzerland. Abstract number 33159.

20. "HIVNET Scientific Steering Committee Group Meeting Summary," July 10-11, 1997. Natcher Center in Bethesda, Maryland.

21. Rob Eder. "Shifting Paradigms: Sexual Revolution Continues to Drive Condom Market Evolution," *Drug Store News*, December 8, 1997, p. CP27.

22. "Women's Health Is Lake's Main Focus; Lake Consumer Products Inc," *Chain Drug Review,* June 23, 1997, p. 64.

23. "University Sees Future for Invisible Condom," *The Orange County Register*, November 14, 1997, p. A9.

24. Joyce Price. "Federal Study of Lubricant Blasted: Agency to Weigh Effect on Gay Men," *The Washington Times*, July 25, 1996, p. A3.

25. Department of Health and Human Services, Centers for Disease Control and Prevention. "FY 1997 Epidemiologic Research Studies of Acquired Immunodeficiency Syndrome (AIDS) and Human Immunodeficiency Virus (HIV) Infection," *Federal Register* 62 (130): 36514-36522 (1997).

26. C.L. Celum, S.R. Tabet, M. Paradise, C. Surawicz, M. Chesney, M. Gross, A.S. Coletti, H. Brar, T. Elliott, T. Fleming, et al. "Safety, Acceptability, and Biologic Effects of Nonoxynol-9 as a Rectal Microbicide," Abstract presented at ISSTDR in Seville, Spain in October 1997.

27. R.F. Lago, L.H. Harrison, and M. Schechter. "Willingness of participants in an HIV seroincidence study in Rio de Janeiro, Brazil to participate in future vaccine trials," *International Conference on AIDS, July 7-12, 1996* 11(2): 457 (abstract number Pub.C.1119).

28. *A Call for New Methods to Prevent HIV and STDs* pamphlet (Berkeley, CA: Microbicides as an Alternative Solution, 1998).

Chapter 4

1. Gary R. Cohan. "HIV, Cancer, and Male Pap Smears," *The Advocate,* February 7, 1995, p. 44.

2. *Ibid.*

3. See Beryl A. Koblin, Nancy A. Hessol, Ann G. Zauber, Patricia E. Taylor, Susan P. Buchbinder, Mitchell H. Katz, and Cladd E. Stevens. "Increased Incidence of Cancer Among Homosexual Men, New York City and San Francisco, 1978-1990," *American Journal of Epidemiology* 144(10): 916-923 (1996); Joel M. Palefsky, Elizabeth A. Holly, John Gonzales, Jennifer Berline, Daid K. Ahn, and John S. Greenspan. "Detection of Human Papillomavirus DNA in Anal Intraepithelial Neoplasia and Anal Cancer," *Cancer Research* 51: 1014-1019 (1991).

4. Janet R. Daling, Noel S. Weiss, Larry L. Klopfenstein, Leah H. Cochran, Wong Ho Chow, Richard Daifuku, et al. "Correlates of Homosexual Behavior and the Incidence of Anal Cancer," *Journal of the American Medical Association* 247(14): 1988 (1982). For other studies of a similar nature, see Elizabeth A. Holly, Alice S. Whittemore, Diana A. Aston, David K. Ahn, Brian J. Nickoloff, Jennifer L. Kristiansen, et al. "Anal Cancer Incidence: Genital Warts, Anal Fissure or Fistula, Hemorrhoids, and Smoking," *Journal of the National Cancer Institute* 81(22): 1726-1731 (1989).

5. Charles Hennekens and Julie E. Buring. *Epidemiology in Medicine* (Boston: Little, Brown, and Company, 1987), 17.

6. Daling. "Correlates of Homosexual Beahvior," 1990.

7. Hennekens and Buring, *op. cit.,* p. 18.

8. Janet R. Daling, Noel S. Weiss, T. Gregory Hislop, Christopher Maden, Ralph J. Coates, Karen J. Sherman, Rhoda L. Ashley, Marjorie Beagrie, John A. Ryan, and Lawrence Corey. "Sexual Practices, Sexually Transmitted Diseases, and the Incidence of Anal Cancer," *The New England Journal of Medicine* 317(16): 973 (1987).

9. Hennekens and Buring, *op. cit.,* p. 133.

10. *Ibid.*

11. Daling, "Sexual Practices," 973.

12. *Guide to Clinical Preventive Services: Report of the U.S. Preventive Services Task Force*, Second Edition (Baltimore, MD: Williams and Wilkins, 1996), 108.

13. Joel Palefsky. "HPV-Related Disease in Immunosuppressed Individuals." In Gerd Gross and Geo von Krogh (Eds.). *Human Papillomavirus Infections in Dermatovenereology* (Boca Raton, FL: CRC Press, 1997), 227.

14. See Joel Palefsky and R. Barrasso. "HPV Infection and Disease in Men," *Obstetric and Gynecology Clinics of North America* 23(4): 895-916 (December 23, 1996); Mads Melbye, Joel Palefsky, John Gonzales, Lars P. Ryder, Henrik

Nielsen, Olav Bergmann, Jens Pindborg, and Robert J. Biggar, Issue #2. "Immune Status As a Determinant of Human Papillomavirus Detection and its Association with Anal Epithelial Abnormailities," *International Journal of Cancer* 46(3): 203-206 (1990); Joel Palefsky. "Human Papillomavirus Infection Among HIV-Infected Individuals: Implications for Development of Malignant Tumors," *Hematology / Ontology Clinics of North America* 5(2): 357-370 (1991); and Michael Z. Zhang, Kenneth A. Borchardt, and Zhijiang Li. "Condyloma Acuminatum." In Kenneth A. Borchardt and Michael A. Noble (Eds.). *Sexually Transmitted Diseases: Epidemiology, Pathology, Diagnosis, and Treatment* (New York: CRC Press, 1997), 271-282.

15. Joel Palefsky. "Anal Human Papillomavirus Infection and Anal Cancer in HIV-Positive Individuals: An Emerging Problem," *AIDS* 8(3): 290 (1994).

16. Denny Smith. "HIV and Anal Cancer: Anal Pap Smears, Early Treatment, Recommended for High-Risk Men and Women," *AIDS Treatment News*, July 22, 1994.

17. Leopold G. Koss. "The Attack on the Annual 'Pap Smear,'" *Acta Cytologica* 34(5): 596 (1990). See also Kenneth L. Noller. "When One More Pap Smear Is One Too Many," *Gynecologic Oncology* 67(1): 1-2 (1997); and Nancy Volkers. "Problems and Progress with Pap Smear Screening Reviewed," *Journal of the National Cancer Institute* 84(22): 1694-1695 (1992).

18. "National Institutes of Health Consensus Development Conference Statement on Cervical Cancer," *Gynecologic Oncology* 66(3): 353 (1997).

19. Leslie Hanna. "Human Papillomavirus Infection and Anal Neoplasia," *Bulletin of Experimental Treatments for AIDS*, San Francisco AIDS Foundation, September 1997, p. 19. Reprinted by permission of *Bulletin of Experimental Treatments for AIDS*.

20. Joel Palefsky. Presentation at the 1997 National Lesbian and Gay Health Association conference in Atlanta, GA, July 28, 1997. "High Prevalence and Incidence of Anal Cancer Precursers [sic] in Gay Men: Should We Be Screening?"

21. For more details of this study and its findings, see: Sue J. Goldie, K.M. Kuntz, K.A. Freedberg, M. Welton, M.C. Weinstein, and J.M. Palefsky (1998). "Cost-Effectiveness of Screening for Anal Squamous Intraepithelial Lesions in HIV-Infected Men," poster presentation given at 12th World AIDS Conference in Geneva, Switzerland. Abstract number 22307.

22. See Steven Epstein's book *Impure Science: AIDS, Activism, and the Politics of Knowledge* (Los Angeles: University of California Press, 1996).

23. Palefsky. "Anal Human Papillomavirus Infection and Anal Cancer in HIV-Positive Individuals," *AIDS* 8(3), (1994), p. 291.

24. Terri Kapsalis. *Public Privates: Performing Gynecology from Both Ends of the Speculum* (Durham, NC: Duke University Press, 1997), 6.

25. See Chapter 2 in this book on the subject of gay bowel syndrome for a more thorough discussion of the vagina/rectum comparison.

26. Hanna. The course of treatment, however, is not necessarily quite so analogous. There is no consensus on what treatments, if any, will yield health benefits at different stages of HPV lesion development. See Donald W. Northfelt, Patrick

S. Swift, and Joel M. Palefsky. "Anal Neoplasia: Pathogenesis, Diagnosis, and Management," *Hematology/Oncology Clinics of North America* 10(5): 1177-1187 (1996); and Christina M. Surawicz, Philip Kirby, Cathy Critchlow, James Sayer, Carol Dunphy, and Nancy Kiviat. "Anal Dysplasia in Homosexual Men: Role of Anoscopy and Biopsy," *Gastroenterology* 105(3): 658-666 (1993).

27. Catherine Waldby. *AIDS and the Body Politic: Biomedicine and Sexual Difference* (New York: Routledge, 1996), 110.

28. Tina Posner. "What's in a Smear? Cervical Screening, Medical Signs and Metaphors," *Science As Culture* 2(11): 186 (1991).

29. Shireen S. Rajaram, Jeffrey Hill, Carole Rave, and Benjamin F. Crabtree. "A Biographical Disruption: The Case of an Abnormal Pap Smear," *Health Care for Women International* 18(6): 523 (1997).

30. Posner, *op. cit.,* p. 179.

31. Koss, *op. cit.,* p. 596.

32. Susan Sontag. *Illness As Metaphor;* and *AIDS and its Metaphors* (New York: Anchor Books, 1990), 112.

33. *Ibid.,* 114.

34. *Ibid.,* 115.

35. J.M. Palefsky, E.A. Holly, M.L. Ralston, S.P. Arthur, N. Jay, J.M. Berry, M.M. DaCosta, R. Botts, and T.M. Darragh. (1998). "Anal Squamous Intraepithelial Lesions in HIV-Positive and HIV-Negative Homosexual and Bisexual Men: Prevalence and Risk Factors," *Journal of Acquired Immune Deficiency Syndrome and Human Retrovirology* 17(4): 320-326.

36. See also Risa Denenberg. "I'm Gay, So Why Do I Need a Pap Smear?" *LAP Notes: The Newsletter of the Lesbian AIDS Project at Gay Men's Health Crisis,* Spring 1994, p. 8, for a discussion of lesbian Pap smears.

Chapter 5

1. Other treatments for erectile dysfunction actually recovered some of their market share from losses incurred with Viagra's debut. See the Associated Press article "Viagra Sales Drop," July 23, 1998, and April Adamson, "Honeymoon's Over: Viagra Sales Taper Off," *The Advocate* (Baton Rouge, LA), July 23, 1998, p. 9A.

2. *Ibid.*

3. Lewis Griswold. "Widow Spreads Message About Possible Dangers of Viagra," *The Fresno Bee,* July 23, 1998, p. B1.

4. Herminia Palacio and Mitchell Katz. "Viagra and You," *Bay Area Reporter,* August 6, 1998, pp. 21 and 23. Levels of testosterone and anabolic steroids may be similarly effected, warranting lower does of Viagra. See Zachary Bohdan. "Ups and Downs: Viagra Erects Fears of Deadly Combos with HIV, Party Drugs," *San Francisco Frontiers,* July 16, 1998, p. 14.

5. John Gallagher. "What Goes Up Must Come Down," *The Advocate,* June 23, 1998, pp. 60 and 65.

6. "Gay Medical Association Issues Caution in Use of Viagra by Some Gay Men," press release issued by The Gay and Lesbian Medical Association, April 30, 1998.

7. David Kirby. "Viagra Wants to Be (Taken) Alone," *The New York Times,* May 3, 1998, Section 14, p. 6. Copyright© 1998 by *The New York Times,* Reprinted by permission.

8. Pfizer brochure. "The New Facts of Life: Viagra (Sildenafil Citrate)," 1998.

9. Katharine Road. "Viagra: Story of the Little Blue Wonder," *Belfast News Letter*, July 18, 1998, p. 14.

10. Leslie Goldberg. (August 1998). "Comparative Epidemiology of Erectile Dysfunction (ED) in Gay Men," paper presented at the 8th World Meeting on Impotence Research held in Amsterdam. Abstract number 304.

11. "Society Abusing Medical Marvel," *Sun-Sentinel*, July 20, 1998, p. 14A.

12. Michael T. Risher. "Controlling Viagra-Mania," *The New York Times,* July 20, 1998, p. A15.

13. Peter H. Gott. "Health and Fitness," *Capital*, August 14, 1998, p. B2.

14. See Marilyn Elias. "Pill's Possibilities Excite Women," *USA Today,* July 16, 1998, p. 8D; and "Women Use Viagra for Orgasmic Quick Fix," *The Ottawa Sun,* July 19, 1998, p. S18.

15. Road, *op. cit.,* p. 9A.

16. Pat Flanagan. "Sex Drug Set to Break Bank: Doctor Warns Viagra Might Ruin Health Service," *The Mirror*, July 15, 1998, p. 7.

17. "Patient Instructions for Caverject Sterile Powder," leaflet produced by Pharmacia and Upjohn Company, Kalamazoo, MI, 1997.

18. Greg Lugliani. "Oh, Viagra! An Ode to Daddy's Little Blue Helper," *POZ,* August 1998, p. 70.

19. Karen McAllister and John G. Taylor. "Fresno VA Spurns Viagra Pending a National Ruling; Guidelines Expected Next Month on Impotence Drug," *The Fresno Bee,* June 23, 1998, p. A1.

20. "Playing Doctor: Prescription Proposal Preposterous," *The Montgomery Advertiser,* August 8, 1998, p. 9A; and "Viagra Ban Sought," *AIDS Policy and Law* August 21, 1998, p. 1.

21. "Proposal in Alabama for Viagra Ban," United Press International, August 4, 1998.

22. Lugliani, *op. cit.,* p. 70.

23. See Rafael Diaz. (1997). *Latino Gay Men and HIV: Culture, Sexuality, and Risk Behavior* (New York: Routledge).

24. *Poppers: Can You Afford the Risk?* Brochure produced through Community Substance Abuse Services, San Francisco.

25. Gabriel Rotello. "A Date With Viagra," *The Advocate,* July 7, 1998, p. 72.

26. H.K. Choi, A. Adimoelja, S.C. Kim, D.M. Soebadi, D.H. Seong, R.J. Garceau, et al. "A Dose-Response Study of Alprostadil Sterile Powder (Caverject) for the Treatment of Erectile Dysfunction in Korean and Indonesian Men," *International Journal of Impotence Research* 9(1): 47-51 (1997).

27. M. Godschalk, D. Gheorghiu, J. Chen, P.G. Katz, T. Mulligan, et al., "Long-Term Efficacy of a New Formulation of Prostaglandin E1 As Treatment for Erectile Failure," *Journal of Urology* 155(3): 915-917 (1996).

28. E. Stewart Geary, Theresa E. Dendinger, Fuad S. Freiha, and Thomas Stamey. "Nerve Sparing Radical Prostatectomy: A Different View," *Journal of Neurology* 154(1): 145-149 (July 1995).

29. Gunilla Ojdeby, Anders Claezon, Einar Brekkan, Michael Haggman, and Bo Johan Norlen. "Urinary Impotence and Sexual Impotence After Radical Prostatectomy," *Scandinavian Journal of Urology and Nephrology* 30(6): 473-477 (1996).

30. For more discussion of erectile treatments that are not administered orally with medication, see L. Garcia-Reboll, J.P. Mulhall, and I. Goldstein. "Drugs for the Treatment of Impotence," *Drugs and Aging* 11(2): 140-151 (August 1997).

31. David Saul. "If Men Were Still Men, They Wouldn't Need Viagra," *Toronto Star*, July 21, 1998, p. 5A.

32. *Ibid.*

Index

Page numbers followed by the letter "f" indicate figures; those followed by the letter "t" indicate tables.

Order Your Own Copy of
This Important Book for Your Personal Library!

SMEARING THE QUEER
Medical Bias in the Health Care of Gay Men

_____ in hardbound at $39.95 (ISBN: 0-7890-0410-0)

_____ in softbound at $17.95 (ISBN: 1-56023-926-3)

COST OF BOOKS_____

OUTSIDE USA/CANADA/
MEXICO: ADD 20%_____

POSTAGE & HANDLING_____
(US: $3.00 for first book & $1.25
for each additional book)
Outside US: $4.75 for first book
& $1.75 for each additional book)

SUBTOTAL_____

IN CANADA: ADD 7% GST_____

STATE TAX_____
(NY, OH & MN residents, please
add appropriate local sales tax)

FINAL TOTAL_____
(If paying in Canadian funds,
convert using the current
exchange rate. UNESCO
coupons welcome.)

☐ **BILL ME LATER:** ($5 service charge will be added)
(Bill-me option is good on US/Canada/Mexico orders only;
not good to jobbers, wholesalers, or subscription agencies.)

☐ Check here if billing address is different from
shipping address and attach purchase order and
billing address information.

Signature_____

☐ **PAYMENT ENCLOSED: $**_____

☐ **PLEASE CHARGE TO MY CREDIT CARD.**

☐ Visa   ☐ MasterCard   ☐ AmEx   ☐ Discover
☐ Diner's Club

Account #_____

Exp. Date_____

Signature_____

Prices in US dollars and subject to change without notice.

NAME_____

INSTITUTION_____

ADDRESS_____

CITY_____

STATE/ZIP_____

COUNTRY_____ COUNTY (NY residents only)_____

TEL_____ FAX_____

E-MAIL_____
May we use your e-mail address for confirmations and other types of information? ☐ Yes   ☐ No

Order From Your Local Bookstore or Directly From
The Haworth Press, Inc.
10 Alice Street, Binghamton, New York 13904-1580 • USA
TELEPHONE: 1-800-HAWORTH (1-800-429-6784) / Outside US/Canada: (607) 722-5857
FAX: 1-800-895-0582 / Outside US/Canada: (607) 772-6362
E-mail: getinfo@haworthpressinc.com
PLEASE PHOTOCOPY THIS FORM FOR YOUR PERSONAL USE.

BOF96